Communication Variables

of

Cerebral Palsied

and

Mentally Retarded Children

Communication Variables
of
Cerebral Palsied
and
Mentally Retarded Children

—————————— *By* ——————————

ORVIS C. IRWIN, Ph.D.

Formerly
Professor
Iowa Child Welfare Research Station
University of Iowa
Iowa City, Iowa
and
Professor
Institute of Logopedics
Wichita State University
Wichita, Kansas

With a Foreword by
Dorothea McCarthy
Professor Emeritus
Fordham University
New York, New York

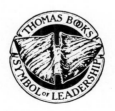

CHARLES C THOMAS • **PUBLISHER**
Springfield • *Illinois* • *U.S.A.*

Published and Distributed Throughout the World by
CHARLES C THOMAS • PUBLISHER
BANNERSTONE HOUSE
301-327 East Lawrence Avenue, Springfield, Illinois, U.S.A.
NATCHEZ PLANTATION HOUSE
735 North Atlantic Boulevard, Fort Lauderdale, Florida, U.S.A.

© *1972, by* CHARLES C THOMAS • PUBLISHER
ISBN 0-398-02322-0
Library of Congress Catalog Card Number: 77-169883

With **THOMAS BOOKS** *careful attention is given to all details of manufacturing and design. It is the Publisher's desire to present books that are satisfactory as to their physical qualities and artistic possibilities and appropriate for their particular use.* **THOMAS BOOKS** *will be true to those laws of quality that assure a good name and good will.*

Printed in the United States of America
EE-11

iv

To Hattie

Foreword

ORVIS C. IRWIN is primarily a scientist who in this volume presents an overwhelming mass of data on the communication skills of cerebral palsied and mentally retarded children. His approach is atomistic for he breaks the communication process down into its basic elements to find valid and reliable measures of each hypothesized element; then he compares large samples of cerebral palsied children with mentally retarded children and also with · normals. His concept of communication goes far beyond the usual articulation and sound discrimination aspects to include relevant psychological functions such as auditory, memory, vocabulary (both understood and actively used) and syntactical features of sentences, as well as anxiety manifested during oral communication. He has mastered the difficult techniques of phonology and holds to high standards of psychometrics in standardizing and sampling, all of which he explains so simply that the statistically unsophisticated reader can appreciate the meaning of his data. With the zeal and dedication of the true scientist, he has gathered an amazing amount of information in systematic fashion, travelling to most states of the union including Hawaii and many Provinces of Canada, examining in detail all the cerebral palsied children he could find (over 1600 in overlapping subgroups). The resulting series of studies presented in this volume is undoubtedly the greatest mass of meticulously gathered information on the communication skills of such a rarely occurring clinical syndrome as the cerebral palsied ever to appear in the literature.

The rigorous criteria which are met methodologically in study after study yield amazingly consistent results which should be of interest to and available for ready reference to speech pathologists, speech therapists and research workers as well as pediatric neurologists, pediatricians and developmental psychologists. All people working in the field of psychology, even if not concerned with cerebral palsied children or speech problems, but those primarily interested in experimental design and seeking help in setting up simple projects for research, would profit greatly from reading several chapters of this volume. These chapters are excellent examples yielding demonstrations of the fertile scientific mind at work setting up model research on question after question, with replication for verification when needed, and bleeding the data for all the facts to be gleaned from the available information.

This book is Irwin's crowning glory showing once again how well deserved was his 1970 G. Stanley Hall Award in Developmental Psychology given by the Division on Developmental Psychology of the American Psychological Association for his outstanding contributions in a lifetime of dedicated research.

DOROTHEA MCCARTHY

Introduction

THIS BOOK BRINGS together in one place the results of a series of studies which were completed over a period of thirteen years. It attempts to collate and organize a number of investigations in the speech and language of speech handicapped children. In this manner their interrelations perhaps may be better presented and their implications the more advantageously apprehended. It does not pretend to be a systematic treatment of the entire area of communication. Rather it is a series of studies initiated by the author's interest in certain problems and variables which he considers to be important in the efforts to communicate by cerebral palsied and mentally retarded children. A theory for organizing, integrating and interpreting the variables will be proposed. It is based on the definitions and nature of the construct (Margenau, 1950).

The variables are (1) articulation, (2) sound discrimination, (3) abstraction, (4) vocabulary, (5) the sentence, (6) immediate memory span and (7) manifest anxiety. There are others but these are among the most crucial. The position held is that the set of seven variables, if taken collectively, constitutes the basic meaning of the phenomenon of communication. The interrelations among the variables and factors affecting them will be treated. In addition a viewpoint defining the phenomenon of communication is provided. The justification for including certain psychological processes under the construct of communication is that this construct includes more than merely structural linguistics. An integral part of it are complex mental activities such as memory, abstraction and discrimination. A final chapter will recapitulate and discuss the more prominent results of the endeavor.

It would be helpful first to consider the concept of the variable. A variable is something, a property or quality, which can take on different values from low to high. Anything to which numbers can be assigned is a variable. It may be defined also as an operationally based construct. It will be used here to explicate the construct of communication. Definitions of the construct will be given presently. A social definition of communication also will be presented and analyzed.

An important consideration relates to the independence of these variables for a treatment of them individually depends on this factor. Although the set of seven variables are all relevant to the concept of communication, they nevertheless may be treated as independent variables. This can be demonstrated statistically. For instance, the coefficient of correlation for articulation and sound discrimination is $r = .21$. Its coefficient of determination is $r^2 = .04$. It follows that the coefficient of nondetermination is .96. This means that there is an absence of relationship in the amount of 96%. This value becomes the estimate of the independence of these two variables.

Articulation and abstraction are correlated with $r = .36$. Then $r^2 = .13$ and the value of nondetermination is 87%. Articulation correlates with the vocabulary of expression $r = .33$. With vocabulary of comprehension $r = .24$. The percents of nondetermination are 89 and 76. Sound discrimination and abstraction correlates $r = .67$, thus $r^2 = .43$ and the degree of independence amounts to 58%. Between sound discrimination and expression $r = .33$ which yields independence in the amount of 89%. The value with comprehension is 76%. Abstraction has a correlation with vocabulary of expression of $r = .47$, with comprehension it is .55, the values for nondetermination being 78% and 63%. These measures are based on the scores of cerebral palsied children.

When the coefficients of nondetermination are derived from the scores of mentally retarded children, they also provide evidence for the independence of the variables. A few instances will be given. The percent of nondetermination between sound discrimination and abstraction is 71; between sound discrimiation and vocabulary it is 81. It is quite evident from these sets of values that the variables are substantially independent.

Obviously in this situation it would be difficult to integrate these discordant variables under the theory of any one of them. Since each variable is largely independent this means that information about one of them gives scant information about the others. This can be illustrated also in terms of the internal structure of language. The theory of distinctive features (Jakobson and Halle, 1957) states that the differences between all the sounds of a language can be accounted for by indicating the presence or absence of distinctive qualities of the sounds. The theory of distinctive features is basic in the study of phonology, but it is useless as a complete theory of the sentence. The theory of partial difference of content applies to the morpheme (Gleason, 1955) but not to the sentence. Transformational grammar with its set of rewrite rules and the phrase marker constitute the theory of the sentence (Chomsky, 1964). It is clearly distinguished from the two aforementioned theories. Thus among linguistic theories also no one of them successfully integrates the others. Moreover it may be remarked that the structural theory of grammar is foreign and inappropriate as an explanation of sound discrimination or articulation or the other variables considered in this book. Since the notion of a single variable cannot be used to unify the whole field of communication, the question then arises regarding what approach is available? It will be shown later that the problem may be solved by considering each variable an independent aspect of an inclusive definition of communication.

It was previously stated that a variable is a symbol to which a distribution of numbers can be allocated. It remains to be shown how this can be done and what operations are necessary to administer the tests. One of the articulation tests used in the investigation includes eighty-seven items, the other is constructed with thirty items. The operations for selecting them will be described later. For the operation of assigning numbers to represent quantities three rules were followed: each correct response is given a score of 1 and each error is 0; the score on the test is equal to the number of items correctly articulated by the subject.

Articulation scores can be related to a number of factors such as chronological and mental ages; the type, degree and extent of palsy; and the right and left hemiplegia. They may be correlated with ratings of general speech ability. The articulation scores of retarded children can be related to biological, psychological and cultural factors—for instance, to age or educational status such as educable and trainable or to various classifications such as borderline, mild, moderate, severe and profound retardation. Cross-relationships with other variables also can be made. There are accordingly a number of ways to process the articulation scores in order to reveal the presence of regularities or laws. Thus it is in terms of operational rules and processing that articulation ultimately is defined and has meaning.

What has been said of articulation holds for the other variables of the set. The operations performed with each test define the meaning of that variable. Furthermore, and this is important, it is held that this set of variables or concepts defines the construct of communication as used in this research. This view will be developed presently.

Communication may be considered from another viewpoint as an aspect of a social situation. Communication is a social event. It is not an adventitious accretion to man's usual activities or his historical development. It is an intrinsic and pervasive instrumentality. It not only promotes ordinary human interpersonal relations, but in a complex and highly technical society it has survival value. It is the major element in the myriad socioeconomic activities which compose the intricate fabric of local, national and international intercourse. Without the apparatus of communication a community would be almost totally disrupted. Without the syntactic structure of speech and its derivatives, we would be reduced to the gestures, cries and sign stage of the lower forms of life.

The social definition of communication, however, can be reconciled and assimilated to a more basic operational approach. To be specific we might consider the concept of communication in the light of two speech variables, namely articulation and sound discrimination. The former refers to verbal output. It is a stimulus variable. Sound discrimination is a response variable. A verbally expressed discrimination represents a response and may be a stimulus also. My articulated speech is a stimulus which evokes a discrimination on your part. Your discrimination response, when expressed, becomes a stimulus to me which in turn evokes a response, and so on. This is obvious and nothing new. The elemental functions of articulation and discrimination constitute an integral part of the communication concept. They are at the base of an understanding of it.

Communication is, however, more than this. It involves content or meaning. Since meaning has many connotations a better term is message. It refers to whatever content or information is being articulated and discriminated. Accordingly, as a first approximation communication may be defined as a social event which can be analyzed in terms of three elements: articulation of sounds, discrimination of sounds and a message. This is the core of the social concept of communication.

This concept, it should be pointed out, has included in its designation two variables, articulation and discrimination, which in turn are defined operationally. It follows, therefore, that the social definition is not primary. It has been converted and reduced to an operational basis. In like manner a word and a sentence when expressed may be considered to be social events. The cognitive processes of abstraction, anxiety and memory are intermediate variables in the social episode. However, their reality is an inferred or postulated "reality." That is, they are constructs. The abilities of discrimination and articulation are inferred from speech responses. Anxiety is postulated from certain manifest behaviors and answers to questions. Other processes such as abstraction and memory also are inferences from test results. These are all constructs, but it should be emphasized that they are operationally defined. It is in this manner that the definition of communication as a social event is subsumed and assimilated in a matrix of operational definitions. The set of variables, taken as a whole, therefore constitutes the definition of the construct of communication.

It may be remarked that the logic of this interpretation is derived from definitions of the construct itself. A construct is a concept which has been deliberately invented (constructed) for a special scientific purpose. There are two types of constructs: constitutive and operational (Kerlinger, 1965; Torgerson, 1958; Margenau, 1950). The constitutive type defines a construct with other constructs or variables. The operational construct assigns meaning by indicating what instructions or activities or operations are needed to measure a variable. In the present discussion each of the seven variables is defined operationally. These operational constructs in turn constitute the definition of the construct of communication. It is in this sense that communication is an instance of the constitutive type of construct. Moreover it is in this manner that the constitutive construct of communication serves as a unifying rubric for the several variables.

Since its status as a constitutive construct means it is tied to data (albeit indirectly via a series of operational definitions), it is invested with the property of verifiability or the requirement of experimental repeatability. Moreover, it has the further property of connectibility. It can be connected to other constitutive and operational constructs. Some of these possibilities are biological concepts such as chronological and mental age and genetic constitution. They are also related to physiological, neural, chemical and anatomical factors including brain damage and palsy. Learning is a construct related to communication and there are pertinent connections with psychiatric and medical constructs. Others to which the construct of communication may be connected are environmental, such as educational, socioeconomic and cultural concepts. The discipline of structural linguistics consists of a complicated cluster of variables each with an independent theory. Phonology, morphology and syntax are operationally defined linguistic constructs which enter into and further define the constitutive construct of communication. The engineering theory of information and its array of constructs concerned with technical equipment can be integrated with this definition of communication. It is quite evident then that the constitutive construct of communication has the characteristic of multiple relations necessary to a science. The requirement of connectibility with other constructs accordingly widens the meaningfulness of the construct.

However this may be, this book primarily is concerned with the data and the operations on which the construct of communication must be founded. Before considering these data, something should be said about the operations employed in collecting them.

STANDARDIZATION OF THE TESTS

It is necessary to explain the theory of test construction from which the series of instruments used in the investigation was developed. The fundamental principle of test construction is that a test must be standardized on samples of the type of population with which ultimately it is to be used. This means for example if a test has been standardized for use with cerebral palsied children, before administering it to mentally retarded cases, it must be restandardized on a sample of mentally retarded children. Obviously the principle holds for the reverse situation as well. The instruments employed in the present investigation were standardized according to this principle.

Three operations were completed for the purpose of constructing the tests. The first concerns the selection and analysis of items to be included. The second procedure relates to the problem of test reliability. The third concerns the validity of the tests.

It may be helpful to describe step by step the operations which were utilized to complete the standardization of the tests. As the first step a pool of possible items was assembled for each test. The author consulted the pertinent literature, word tests and other speech and language tests. He examined children's books and searched through dictionaries and other sources to compile a large pool of items. The pool was then submitted to three speech pathologists who were instructed to select the hundred items which according to their judgment were best adapted to the level of cerebral palsied children, to their general level of understanding. That is, the items were judged for their face validity, their content validity and for construct validity.

Face validity refers to what a test on its surface appears to measure. The test seems to the testee to look valid. Judges were instructed to select items which would not appear to be entirely impossible for the children to respond to. Content validity assures that items constitute pertinent subject matter to the purpose for which the test is to be used. Materials foreign to the field are excluded. Construct validity also is a matter to be determined by the subjective judgment of experts. It is concerned with the basic concept to be measured—that is, with the processes and functions that are applied to some content. Construct or concept validity is an estimate of the psychological, motor or language function or concept which a test should incorporate. This was the judgmental task undertaken by the speech pathologists. It was decided that for an item to be acceptable, the speech pathologists must agree unanimously on it. If one of the judges did not approve an item, it was not included in the list of one hundred. It should be noted that these hundred items were selected essentially on the basis of subjective judgments. This set then constituted the preliminary form of the test.

However, it is also necessary to subject the items selected by the judges to a more objective treatment. Accordingly the preliminary test was taken out to speech centers in several states and administered to other groups of cerebral palsied children. Incidentally, this procedure accords with the aim of the investigation to base the tests on nationwide samples. The next step was to process these data in a statistical item analysis. The item analysis was conducted according to three criteria: the difficulties of the items for cerebral palsied children, their uniqueness and the discriminating power of the item.

The difficulty of an item is determined by the percentage of testees who succeed in passing it. If a large percentage succeed on an item it is considered to be easy. The smaller percentage which pass it, the more difficult it must be. An ideal range of items difficulty is approximately 15% or 20% to 85% or 90%. If an item falls within this range, it may be incorporated in the final form of the test.

Whereas the concept of difficulty is in terms of items, discriminating power refers to the subjects who take the test. This means that the items should discriminate among the testees. There should be a range of scores among the subjects for if all of them made the same score on an item it would lack discriminating power. This criterion is determined by means of a coefficient of correlation. A convenient shortcut is provided by Flanagan's table of values of product moment coefficients of correlation (1939). The coefficients of discriminating power should be fairly high. In general they should exceed $r = .50$. Since the correlation is between item values and the whole test taken as an external criterion, discriminating power may also be considered to be a measure of item validity.

Uniqueness of an item refers to the nonduplication of functions among the items. If two items correlate strongly, presumably they are performing the same function in a test. Accordingly one of them may be discarded. The statistical criterion of uniqueness is that the intercorrelations among the items must be low, in general below the cutting point r = .50. The phi coefficient of correlation may be used to determine this criterion. The principle of uniqueness provides for economy in the administration of a test. A further criterion follows from the above statements. It concerns the relation between the coefficients of discriminating power and those of uniqueness. The values of the former, in the main, should be higher than those of the latter.

In summary the difficulty criterion provides that items are adapted to the abilities of the testees. That is, it provides confirmation of face, content and construct validity of the test. Discriminating power assures the validity of the separate items and discriminates the subjects. Uniqueness makes it reasonably certain that the test administratively is an economical instrument. It is in this manner that the item analysis completes and reinforces objectively the subjective judgments of the speech pathologists who made the original selection of the items.

After the item analysis of the test was completed, the procedure was to take it out in its revised form to another set of states and administer it to samples of children in a number of speech centers. The data were brought back and the tests were evaluated for their reliability and validity.

Before taking up the problem of test reliability, an evaluation was made of observer reliability. A research stands or falls on the reliability of the observer who conducts the experiment. The question is, How can the dependability of the sense data or percepts of an observer be established? In this work the reader of the tape record needs to be checked. The procedure was to have two or more readers or observers record their observations simultaneously but independently. If the correlation between the independent sets of observations is high or if the percent of agreement is substantial, observer reliability may be accepted.

By the same token, the percent of disagreement will be a measure of the amount of observer unreliability.

Test reliability may be defined generally as the internal consistency of the data of an experiment. If one part of a body of data confirms another part, the consistency is taken as the criterion of reliability. This principle underlies the split half method. Reliability of the present tests usually was determined by means of a Kuder-Richardson formula No. 20 (1937) which is a refinement of the split half method. Moreover replications frequently were made in various parts of the country. In this fashion substantial checks on the reliability of test results were made.

Several statistical procedures were employed: (1) if the means of administrations of a test to different samples of cases are not significantly different and if the variances are homogeneous, reliability may be considered to be adequate; (2) with repeated administrations of a test to the same sample of subjects, reliability will be substantial if the means are alike, if the variances are not significantly different and if the correlation is high; and (3) if the means of two tests administered to the same sample of children are the same, if the variances are homogeneous and if the correlation is substantial, parallel form reliability will be satisfactorily achieved. These several methods for establishing reliability were employed in these studies.

The problem of the validity of these tests also needs consideration. In addition to face and construct validity as well as item validity, the validity of each test as a whole was determined. In some instances the studies have made use of validity coefficients with other accepted standardized tests. Correlations also were calculated with external criteria, such as medical evaluations, or with teachers or therapists ratings of general speech ability and intelligibility, or with chronological or mental age. A method frequently depended on in these studies is the method of extreme groups (Anastasi, 1955; Adkins, 1947). If the individuals who have taken a speech test can be classified according to an external criterion, the means of the speech scores of the extremes of that distribution may be compared. If the application of the statistic reveals that the difference is significant the result may be accepted as evidence of validity. For example if the articulation scores of an older chronological age group are significantly different from those of a younger age group, presumably the articulation test may be accepted as valid. Throughout this research alpha was set at the .05 level.

Attention should be called to an anomalous situation. It is not impossible that a validity coefficient of correlation may be low, but that an application of an analysis of variance or a test to extreme groups still may indicate a significant trend or difference. This situation has occasionally been encountered provided the r is not below .25.

Most of the studies reported here were standardized using the 5% criteria outlined above.

ADMINISTRATION OF THE TESTS

The subjects of these studies include cerebral palsied and mentally retarded children and also some aphasic and functional cases. Groups of nonafflicted children in elementary school grades were tested for comparative or control purposes. In each study a detailed description of the children is provided.

A number of conditions should be controlled during the testing period. When the child is brought to the examining room, he should be seated facing the examiner who sits with his face in a good light. Considerable effort should be made to put the child at ease. This will of course vary with the individual. The instructions to the subjects are simple, but the tester should speak slowly and clearly and should be careful that the child attends to the task. The time taken by the child is of no importance. These are power, not speed, tests.

The tests are short. The reason for this lies in the fact that these children fatigue easily and their attention span is brief. Occasionally it may be necessary not to give a test in its entirety at one sitting. Moreover it is well to remember that cerebral palsied children differ widely in their personalities and behavior. Some are extremely passive while others may fling themselves about wildly. Many will respond promptly, others are shy and have great difficulty in the sheer utterance of sounds and words. These cases will delay inordinately. There are a few who even anticipate the stimulus and attempt to overrun the completion of it. Quite a few will give a neutral response. The therapist will do well to be aware of the differences among the children and adjust the rate of the examination patiently to the needs of the child. Care is exercised to eliminate cases with questionable hearing. Audiometric tests are administered.

Finally, it may be useful to indicate that in the treatment of the problems reported a threefold pattern of organization generally was followed. The first is a consideration of the construction of the test. The second is a general treatment of the status of the particular test results including an analysis of the factors relating to the problem. Thirdly, a consideration and analysis of errors present in the test results is presented. This is illustrated in the first three units which deal with a set of front consonants. The first unit describes a short test, the second is an analysis of the status of five consonants in the speech of the children, and the third is a treatment of substitution and omission errors in the speech of cerebral palsied children. This pattern will be followed whenever feasible. In a couple of instances this pattern has been abbreviated because the research has been discontinued with the author's retirement.

In order to save space and reduce redundancy, many original tables have been eliminated. If the reader cares to see them, they are found in the original reports. Their substance, however, have been indicated in the body of the text. Tables which present essential data have been retained.

A description of the subjects for each of the studies is found in the Appendix.

Finally, it is hoped that the findings and the viewpoint presented in this book may prove to be of value to the speech scientist. Moreover, it is hoped that they will contribute to the practice of the clinician and therapist, for successful clinical practice depends ultimately on basic research. These studies on several communication variables should provide the clinician with fundamental knowledge concerning important aspects of the speech of cerebral palsied and mentally retarded patients. With this information before him, it may be assumed that the therapist's evaluation and understanding of the problem of the speech deviate child may be further clarified and enhanced.

An application to the practical therapy situation of the data contained in this volume has been made in detail by means of a series of percentile curves, grids and profiles (Irwin, 1970). These diagnostic devices are intended to be used to secure a complete and easily read picture of the communication problems of the handicapped child.

Acknowledgments

IT WOULD BE impossible to list all the names of the several hundred therapists, teachers, speech pathologists, parents, pediatricians, psychologists, directors of speech centers and hospital schools, and supervisors of special education in all parts of the country, in Canada and Hawaii, who have cooperated willingly and unreservedly to promote this research project. To them I express my deepest appreciation and gratitude. I especially want to thank Dr. Boyd R. McCandless, former Director of the Iowa Child Welfare Research Station, who assisted in the initiation of the project. Dr. Martin F. Palmer, Director of the Institute of Logopedics, made it possible to continue the project after my retirement at the University of Iowa. Its success depended in large measure on Mrs. Don Leamon, secretary, who patiently and efficiently assisted in the monotonous clerical work and the calculations. I also want to acknowledge the help of my son, Don A. Irwin, who read the manuscript and made useful suggestions. It would be impossible for me to adequately acknowledge the invaluable cooperation of the five assistants who contributed a considerable part of the project. They are Pura M. Flores, Ph.D.; Donald D. Hammill, Ed.D.; Dale O. Irwin, Ph.D.; Paul J. Jensen, Ph.D.; and Joseph W. Korst, M.A. I am deeply indebted to them.

Without the financial aid of the National Institute of Neurological Diseases and Blindness, U.S. Public Health Service, this research could not have been conducted on a nationwide basis.

Wichita   ORVIS C. IRWIN

CONTENTS

Page

Foreword—DOROTHEA McCARTHY vii

Introduction ix

Acknowledgments xxiii

PART I

ARTICULATION

Chapter

1. A SHORT TEST FOR USE WITH CEREBRAL PALSIED CHILDREN . .   5
2. STATUS OF FIVE FRONT CONSONANTS IN THE SPEECH OF
   CEREBRAL PALSIED CHILDREN   10
3. SUBSTITUTION AND OMISSION ERRORS   16
4. A SECOND SHORT TEST   18
5. VALIDATION OF SHORT CONSONANT ARTICULATION TESTS ...   22
6. A THIRD SHORT CONSONANT TEST   25
7. CORRECT STATUS OF A THIRD SET OF CONSONANTS   28
8. A FOURTH SHORT CONSONANT TEST   34
9. RESTANDARDIZATION OF THE TEMPLIN INITIAL DOUBLE
   CONSONANT BLEND TEST   37
10. CORRECT STATUS OF INITIAL DOUBLE CONSONANT BLENDS   42
11. SUBSTITUTIONS AND OMISSIONS OF INITIAL DOUBLE
    CONSONANT BLENDS   48
12. A TEST OF FINAL DOUBLE CONSONANT BLENDS   52
13. CORRECT STATUS OF FINAL DOUBLE CONSONANT BLENDS   57
14. SUBSTITUTIONS AND OMISSIONS OF FINAL DOUBLE
    CONSONANT BLENDS   62
15. STANDARDIZATION OF A TEST OF FINAL DOUBLE
    REVERSED CONSONANT BLENDS   66
16. STATUS OF ARTICULATION OF FINAL REVERSED
    CONSONANT BLENDS   69
17. A TEST OF TRIPLE CONSONANT BLENDS   73
18. A SHORT VOWEL TEST   77
19. CORRECT STATUS OF VOWELS IN THE SPEECH OF CHILDREN
    WITH CEREBRAL PALSY   81
20. A SHORT DIPHTHONG TEST   85
21. CORRECT STATUS OF DIPHTHONGS   89
22. REPLICATION OF AN INVESTIGATION OF DIPHTHONGS
    ARTICULATION   92

Chapter   *Page*

23. SPEECH DIFFERENCES AMONG CEREBRAL PALSIED SUBCLASSES . .   95
24. AN INTEGRATED ARTICULATION TEST   99
25. DIFFICULTIES OF CONSONANT SOUNDS   109
26. DIFFICULTIES OF CONSONANT SOUNDS IN TERMS OF
    MANNER, PLACE AND VOICING   112
27. THE APPLICABILITY OF AN ARTICULATION TEST WITH
    MENTALLY RETARDED CHILDREN   123
28. A SHORT ARTICULATION TEST FOR USE WITH MENTALLY
    RETARDED CHILDREN   129
29. REPLICATION OF THE SHORT ARTICULATION TEST WITH
    CEREBRAL PALSIED CHILDREN   136
30. CORRECT ARTICULATION OF TEN DIFFICULT CONSONANTS
    BY CHILDREN WITH CEREBRAL PALSY   142
31. COMPARISON OF ARTICULATION SCORES OF CEREBRAL
    PALSIED AND MENTALLY RETARDED CHILDREN   146
32. A SECOND COMPARATIVE STUDY OF ARTICULATION OF CERE-
    BRAL PALSIED AND MENTALLY RETARDED CHILDREN   151
33. THE RELATION OF A SHORT TO A LONG CONSONANT TEST   155

PART II
SOUND DISCRIMINATION

34. A TEST OF SOUND DISCRIMINATION   159
35. A PARALLEL TEST OF SOUND DISCRIMINATION   170
36. A COMPARISON OF SOUND DISCRIMINATION OF MENTALLY
    RETARDED AND CEREBRAL PALSIED CHILDREN   177
37. AN ITEM ANALYSIS OF A SOUND DISCRIMINATION TEST OF
    MENTALLY RETARDED CHILDREN   183

PART III
ABSTRACTION

38. AN ABSTRACTION TEST   191
39. SOME RESULTS WITH AN ABSTRACTION TEST   200
40. AN ABSTRACTION TEST ADAPTED FOR USE WITH MENTALLY
    RETARDED CHILDREN   203

PART IV
VOCABULARY

41. WORD EQUIPMENT OF SPASTIC AND ATHETOID CHILDREN   211
42. A COMPARISON OF THE VOCABULARIES OF USE AND
    OF UNDERSTANDING   214
43. VOCABULARY ABILITY OF TWO SAMPLES OF CEREBRAL
    PALSIED CHILDREN   222
44. THE RELATION OF VOCABULARIES OF USE AND UNDERSTAND-
    ING TO SEVERAL VARIABLES   224
45. A COMPARISON OF THE VOCABULARIES OF USE AND OF
    UNDERSTANDING BY MENTALLY RETARDED CHILDREN   228

Chapter *Page*

PART V
SENTENCE

46. LENGTH OF DECLARATIVE SENTENCES 237
47. NUMBER AND LENGTH OF SENTENCES IN THE LANGUAGE
OF MENTALLY RETARDED CHILDREN 241

PART VI
MEMORY SPAN

48. IMMEDIATE MEMORY SPAN OF MENTALLY RETARDED
CHILDREN 249
49. VERBAL AND NUMERICAL IMMEDIATE MEMORY SPANS OF
MENTALLY RETARDED CHILDREN 252
50. RELATIONS AMONG MEASURES OF THE IMMEDIATE
MEMORY SPAN 258

PART VII
ANXIETY

51. A MANIFEST ANXIETY SCALE FOR USE WITH CEREBRAL
PALSIED CHILDREN 265

PART VIII
LANGUAGE

52. A LANGUAGE TEST 271
53. REPLICATIONS AND RELIABILITY OF FOUR SPEECH TESTS 277
54. SUMMARY OF RELIABILITY COEFFICIENTS OF SIX SPEECH
TESTS FOR USE WITH HANDICAPPED CHILDREN 279
55. CORRELATIONS OF FIVE SPEECH TESTS AND THE
WISC VERBAL SCALE 283
56. REGIONAL AND SEX DIFFERENCES IN THE LANGUAGE OF
CEREBRAL PALSIED CHILDREN ON FIVE SPEECH TESTS 287
57. COMPARISON OF SCORES OF CEREBRAL PALSIED, SUBNORMAL
AND NORMAL CHILDREN ON FIVE SPEECH TESTS 290
58. RECAPITULATION AND DISCUSSION 294

PART IX
APPENDIX

A. *Description of Subjects* 317
B. *Charts* 337
C. *Record Forms* 349

PART X
BIBLIOGRAPHY

Bibliography 359
Author Index 367
Subject Index 369

Communication Variables

of

Cerebral Palsied

and

Mentally Retarded Children

PART I

ARTICULATION

The important part which articulation plays in the act of communication was indicated in the Introduction. Its importance is attested by the extended space devoted to it in this volume. Articulation is the initiatory or stimulus phase of the conversation episode. A further reason for its significance consists in the fact that the substitution or omission of a sound or phoneme in a word decidedly alters the meaning of the word, or the distortion of the sound may render the message unintelligible. The basic function of a phoneme, therefore, is to signal semantic distinctiveness. By substituting p for s in "sin," the word "pin" results. By omitting s in "spin," "pin" is pronounced. We were interested in learning how the cerebral palsied child handles problems of articulation and what his deficiencies are.

The view should be kept in mind that the variable of articulation is considered to be an operational construct which with other variables may be used to define communication as a constitutive construct. This section will analyze the data on articulation in order to reveal its function as an operational construct.

Chapter 1

A Short Test for Use with Cerebral Palsied Children

IN VIEW OF the fact that the administration of extended speech tests is burdensome and fatiguing for cerebral palsied children, the advisability of using short tests needs investigation. It is important for the speech therapist to know to what extent a test composed of a few items is adequate. The present study concerns the construction of a test of five front consonants.

PROCEDURE

In a study of ninety-six cerebral palsied children from 4 to 16 years of age, tape recordings were made of their articulations of five consonantal sounds each in the initial, medial and final positions in fifteen words. The five consonants are *p, b, m, d* and *t* (see Chart 1 in the Appendix). The words were presented in two ways: (1) in the form of pictures to which the children were instructed to respond with the corresponding names and (2) as spoken by the experimenter with the request to repeat the words. All subjects received both kinds of stimulation. A broad transcription of the International Phonetic Alphabet (Fairbanks, 1940) was used in these studies.

There are five criteria by which the usefulness of a test may be judged. They are (1) its reliability, (2) the relative difficulty of the items composing it, (3) the discriminating power or diagnostic value of the items, (4) their uniqueness and (5) the validity of this test. Validity of this test is treated in a separate report. The definitions of these five terms were given in the Introduction.

In this study, the analyses of reliability were made by means of the Kuder-Richardson formula No. 20 (1937). Each correct item in the test receives a credit of one. Therefore, a score equals

5

the number of items to which the subject responds correctly. The Hoyt technique (1941), which estimates test reliability by analysis of variance, also was used.

Discriminating power of an item is determined by its correlation with the whole test. With these data, the discriminating power was secured by means of Flanagan's table of product moment correlations (1939). Uniqueness of items is calculated by their intercorrelations.

RESULTS

Since each of the five consonants appears in the three positions in words, the two tests each were broken down for a preliminary analysis into three subtests, or six subtests in all. To determine the reliabilities of these six subtests the Kuder-Richardson formula was used. The coefficients of reliability calculated by means of this formula range from .74 to .87.

It will be noted in Table 1 that for both the picture and verbal test the values are highest for the initial position.

When the scores for the initial, medial and final positions are pooled for the picture test or the verbal test, the *rs* should be larger. Hoyt's (1941) formula for the coefficient of reliability which can be applied to each set of such pooled scores was used. The formula is

$$r_{xx} = \frac{\sigma^2 \text{ between subjects} - \sigma^2 \text{ residuals}}{\sigma^2 \text{ between subjects}}$$

The analysis of variance of the pooled picture test scores gives a coefficient of reliability of .92. The value for the pooled verbal test is .91. These are reasonably high coefficients.

The difficulties of the five consonants in the speech of cerebral palsied children are recorded in Table 2.

The overall range is from 33% to 88%, the median being 69%.

TABLE 1
Reliability Correlations for Each of Six Subtests

Position	Pictures	Words
Initial	.87	.84
Medial	.74	.79
Final	.81	.79

TABLE 2
Order of Difficulty of Five Consonants in Terms of Percentages

	Position	
Initial	*Medial*	*Final*
p 78	t 33	b 47
t 81	d 67	t 48
b 83	p 71	d 52
m 86	m 71	m 53
d 88	b 72	p 65
Mean 83.2%	62.8%	53.0%

This is an acceptable range. It means that 33% represents the most difficult item and 88% the easiest for the sample of ninety-six cases. Table 2 also indicates that the five sounds are easiest for these subjects in the initial position and are most difficult in the final position. The mean percent values are 83.2% for the initial, 62.8% for the medial, and 53.0% for the final position. A particularly interesting finding is that there is a different order of difficulty for each of these three positions. For instance, *p* is the most difficult item in the initial position and the easiest in the final. It is of medium difficulty in the medial position.

The discriminating power of both the picture and verbal parts of the test is indicated in Table 3 by the correlations of each of the items with the whole test. The initial, medial and final positions are given separately. It is evident that the discriminating power of these five consonants is fairly high. The median coefficient is .75. The range is from .40 to .87. Since the discriminating powers of these items are determined by correlating each of them with the whole test taken as an external criterion, the validity of these five items is established. In other words, discriminating power of an item is equivalent to its validity.

TABLE 3
Discriminating Power of Five Consonants in Three Positions

	Picture Test			Verbal Test		
	Initial	*Medial*	*Final*	*Initial*	*Medial*	*Final*
p	.80	.87	.82	.69	.68	.83
b	.76	.78	.87	.63	.72	.63
m	.71	.78	.86	.53	.40	.83
d	.69	.74	.81	.63	.61	.83
t	.79	.82	.70	.69	.76	.59

TABLE 4
Phi Coefficients of Consonantal Items for the Picture Test

p	b	m	d	t
I	.58	.60	.45	.69
P M	.50	.40	.39	.30
F	.52	.47	.47	.42
I		.56	.56	.55
b M		.49	.33	.42
F		.48	.48	.27
I			.47	.72
m M			.28	.27
F			.67	.34
I				.57
d M				.31
F				.51

In regard to the uniqueness of items, the intercorrelations of the consonant items for the picture test is given in Table 4 and for the verbal test in Table 5.

For the picture test, the phi coefficients run from .27 to .72 with a median of .47; for the verbal test, the range is from .26 to .66 with a median of .47. The value of .75 for the discriminating power is to be contrasted with that of .47 for uniqueness.

It is evident, then, that these short tests adequately meet the four criteria of a useful instrument. The validity of this test will be reported later.

TABLE 5
Phi Coefficients of Consonantal Items for the Verbal Test

p	b	m	d	t
I	.41	.34	.38	.46
P M	.35	.42	.35	.48
F	.63	.51	.52	.32
I		.60	.66	.66
b M		.54	.40	.43
F		.35	.49	.26
I			.57	.60
m M			.38	.49
F			.57	.28
I				.53
d M				.55
F				.37

SUMMARY

A short test of five consonants incorporated in a list of fifteen words was given to ninety-six cerebral palsied children from 4 to 16 years of age. The consonants are *p, b, m, d* and *t*. The study concerns the construction of a short test consisting of five front consonants. Four criteria for the usefulness of a testing instrument are considered. They are (1) its reliability, (2) the difficulty of the item, (3) their discriminating power, (4) their unique-ness and (5) and validity of the test. The coefficients of reliability for the verbal part of the test was .91, for the picture test it was .92. The difficulties of the items ranged from 33% to 88%. The discriminating power of the items was high, the median coefficient being .75, whereas the uniqueness of the items had a median coefficient of .47. Thus this instrument meets four essential criteria of a standardized test and it is reasonable to assume that its use with cerebral palsied children is feasible.

Chapter 2

Status of Five Front Consonants in the Speech of Cerebral Palsied Children

THIS CHAPTER is concerned with the status of articulation by cerebral palsied children of five front consonants as elicited by pictorial and verbal stimulations.

The study was made in an attempt to answer the following questions; Does the kind of stimulation affect the correct consonantal articulation, and if so, in what position in the word pattern do the effects occur? Does the order of stimulation affect the mean number of responses? Do differences exist in the articulation of these consonants in the initial, medial and final positions in words? Are there differences among several schools located in different states? Is there a significant interaction among the factors of stimulation, order of stimulation, position and schools?

PROCEDURE

The study is limited to front consonants and includes three labial sounds *p, b* and *m* and the dentals *t* and *d*. The consonants were presented singly instead of in blends.

Words used in the test were judged by three speech therapists as suitable for research purposes since the words were names of objects, animals and people with which these children ordinarily were acquainted. The items were arranged in random order and this sequence was followed in administering both the pictorial and verbal stimulations. Outline pictures were taken from Utley's (1950) series, a widely used set of pictures. They were selected to illustrate the words. These outlines constitute the picture test and the list of words constitutes the verbal test.

Note: This study was conducted and written with the collaboration of Pura M. Flores, Ph.D.

The test consisted of fifteen pictures and fifteen words. A preliminary word and a preliminary picture in the test were used as trial items. Their purpose was to indicate that the child understood the instructions. The word list is found in Chart 1 in the Appendix.

The five consonantal sounds were each tested in the initial, medial and final positions in the words. An alternate set of items was prepared in case a child failed to perceive an item of the main set.

By means of a table of random numbers, the children in each school were divided into two groups. Both groups received all treatments but the presentation of stimulation was reversed; that is, one group received the picture stimuli first and the verbal stimuli last. The other group received the verbal stimuli first and the pictoral stimuli last. For no child was there a longer time interval than three days nor a shorter interval than one day which separated the administration of the picture stimuli from the verbal stimuli.

The subject was brought to an isolated room and seated before a microphone and the tape recorder was started. Pertinent information about each child was recorded before the test was given. The examiner's instructions to the subject and the subject's responses to the test items were recorded on the tape.

The picture test started with the experimenter giving the following instructions: "I am going to show you some pictures. Will you please give me the name of each picture? Do you understand?" In order to verify if the child understood the nature of the task, a preliminary picture was presented. Before each picture was shown, its number was recorded so that no confusion would arise when the tape was heard later. In no instance during the picture series was a child given a verbal pattern of the word response to imitate.

The procedure was followed during the administration of the verbal stimulation series except for the fact that the subject was asked to repeat each word in imitation of the experimenter's utterance of the word.

RESULTS

There are five measures which lend themselves to the purpose of analyzing the speech sound status of cerebral palsied children. They are the number of correct articulations, substitutions, omissions, no responses and neutral responses. In order that the two observers might have a common basis for judging into which category a response should be classified, the meaning of each category was clarified. The following definitions were adopted: a correct consonantal element is one which is in standard position according to *A Pronouncing Dictionary of American English* (Kenyon and Knott, 1951), a substituted consonantal element is one which is replaced by another consonant, an omitted consonantal element is one which is not articulated in the correct position in response to the stimulus, no response means that no vocalization has occurred, and a neutral response is one which does not resemble the stimulus.

The use of the term "neutral" as a category needs further explanation. In some instances the child will respond either with an entirely different word than the one requested or with a meaningless sound pattern. In either case, there is no resemblance to the word stimulus nor are the consonants present. The neutral category is a catchall category for a response which cannot be classified in one of the other measures.

The present study is limited to an analysis of correct articulations.

In order to study and evaluate the effects of the experimental factors involved in the present study, an analysis of variance of the data was done. The design utilized for this analysis contained four factors. The first two, A and B, were used as Latin square factors, by which the type of stimulation was counterbalanced with the rank order in which the stimulations were presented. The A factor consisted of P picture stimulation and V verbal stimulation. The B factor consisted of (B_1) Order$_1$ and (B_2) Order$_2$. The design also consisted of a "within" factor C for position of the consonant in word patterns. The C factor consisted of I, initial position; M, medial position; and F, final position. The fourth experimental factor was a "between" factor D for school where D_1 represents Iowa Hospital School; D_2, Dowling in Minneapolis; and D_3, Jamestown School in North Dakota.

It is necessary to clarify and to precisely define the term "order" as it will be used in the study. The question here to be investigated is, What is the effect of administering the first sets of stimuli as against the second sets of stimuli? "First" refers to the combination of the pictorial set of stimuli administered first to one group with the verbal set administered first to the other group. "Second" means the combination of the second pictorial administration with the second verbal administration. It is in this sense that the term "order" is used. To repeat, to investigate the main effect of the first stimuli as against second stimuli we paired both firsts and also paired both seconds presentations of stimulations.

The summary for the analysis of variance is presented in Table 6. From the summary table, it will be seen that all higher order interactions are nonsignificant. All interactions with the B factor

TABLE 6

Summary of Analysis of Variance for a Design Consisting of Two Latin Square Factors A and B, a "Within" Factor C and a "Between" Factor D

Source	df	ss	ms	F	p
Between Subjects	95	1101.66			
D (Schools)	2	191.68	95.84	9.83	.001
AB (b) Group	1	16.00	16.00	1.64	nonsig.
AB (b) D (Group by Schools)	2	16.13	8.07		nonsig.
error (b)	90	877.85	9.75		
Within Subjects	480	686.34			
A (Stimulation)	1	9.50	9.50	10.00	.005
B (Order)	1	.45	.45		nonsig.
C (Position)	2	255.44	127.72	109.16	.001
AC (Stimulation by Position)	2	9.11	4.55	9.48	.001
BC (Order by Position)	2	.15	.075		nonsig.
AD (Stimulation by School)	2	2.64	1.32	1.39	nonsig.
BD (Order by School)	2	.64	.32		nonsig.
CD (Position by School)	4	7.05	1.76	1.50	nonsig.
AB (b) C (Grp. by Position)	2	4.19	2.09	1.79	nonsig.
ACD (Stim. by pos. by Sch.)	4	2.23	.56	1.17	nonsig.
BCD (Order by Pos. by Sch.)	4	2.72	.68	1.42	nonsig.
AB (b) CD (Grp. by Pos. by Sch.)	4	8.60	2.15	1.84	nonsig.
Error (w)	450	383.61			
error$_1$ (w)	90	85.77	.95		
error$_2$ (w)	180	211.06	1.17		
error$_3$ (w)	180	86.78	.48		
Total	575	1788.00			

(Order), D factor (schools) and AB (b) groups, are non-significant. The only interaction that is significant is the AC interaction (Stimulation by Position). The main effects of A (Stimulation), C (Position) and D (Schools) are significant. Thus, the null hypotheses of no difference for the pictorial and verbal stimulations, for the initial, medial and final positions and for Iowa, Dowling, and Jamestown schools, may be rejected.

Thus, statistical evidence by means of an analysis of variance was found for rejecting the overall null hypotheses regarding the main effects of position and schools and the interaction effects of stimulation by position. The next task was to apply the t-test to determine whether the null hypotheses could be rejected for each of the pairs of treatments.

The pairs of treatment for the test for position are (1) initial and medial, (2) initial and final and (3) medial and final positions. A further application of the t-test was made comparing the pictorial and verbal stimulations in the (1) initial, (2) medial and (3) final positions. The null hypothesis of no difference concerning three pairs of schools tested. The pairs of schools are (1) Iowa and Dowling, (2) Iowa and Jamestown and (3) Jamestown and Dowling. In the analysis of schools, positions and stimulations were neglected because schools were not found in the main analysis to interact with the factors.

Table 7 shows the means for the initial, medial and final positions. The significance of the differences of the three pairs of positions was tested using a formula to find the critical difference. The critical value of t at the 1% level for 180 degrees of freedom (df) is 2.58. Substituting the values in the formula a critical difference of .40 is obtained. All of the differences exceed the value of .40 and therefore the null hypotheses of no difference between initial and medial, initial and final, and medial and final positions are rejected. The means for the pictorial and the verbal

TABLE 7
Means for the Three Consonantal Positions

Position	Total	N	Mean
Initial	814	96	8.48
Medial	667	96	6.95
Final	501	96	5.22

TABLE 8
Means for Stimuli in Three Positions

	Pictorial			Verbal		
	Total	*N*	*Mean*	*Total*	*N*	*Mean*
Initial	398	96	4.14	416	96	4.33
Medial	305	96	3.18	362	96	3.77
Final	251	96	2.61	250	96	2.60

stimulations in the initial, medial and final positions are presented in Table 8.

A formula for computing the critical difference was used and the value found was .36. It was found that the only value among the differences of means that exceed the critical difference of .36 was the difference between the picture and verbal stimulation in the medial position. Thus, the null hypothesis of no difference may be rejected for only one of the three pairs—that is, the picture and verbal stimulation in the medial position. The differences between the picture and verbal stimulations in the initial and final positions were both nonsignificant and thus the null hypothesis of no difference was retained for these two pairs.

CONCLUSIONS

The pictorial and verbal stimulations have the same effects in the initial and final positions of consonants in word patterns. The verbal stimulation elicits more correct responses in the medial position than does the pictorial stimulation in the same position. Order of the presentation of the stimuli does not affect the number of correct articulations. There are significant differences between the initial and medial positions, initial and final positions, and medial and final positions. Rank order in ease of productions according to position was initial, medial and final position. None of the lower interactions which involve schools, groups and order is significant. None of the higher-order interactions which involve group, order and schools is significant.

Chapter 3

Substitution and Omission Errors

IN A STUDY of the speech sounds of 204 normal preschool children, Wellman, Case, Mengert and Bradbury (1931) found that substitution errors occurred most frequently. Roe and Milisen (1942) observed that substitutions exceeded omissions in the speech of 1,989 children, grade one through grade six. The problem investigated here is whether a similar result obtains with children having cerebral palsy.

PROCEDURE

The subjects were ninety-six children with cerebral palsy ranging in age from 4 to 16 years in the states of Minnesota, North Dakota and Iowa. There were thirty-two from each state. The tests were used in the study, one composed of pictures and the other, a verbal test based on fifteen items involving the five consonants: *p, b, m, d* and *t*.

RESULTS

Table 9 gives the means of the scores for each of the three groups for three categories—correct pronunciation, substitutions and omissions. It is apparent that the means for correct pronunciations are greatly in excess of the means for substitutions and omissions and that the means for omissions are larger than those for substitutions. The next task is to determine if the differences

TABLE 9
Mean Scores for Correct, Substituted and Omitted Consonants

States	N	Correct	Substituted	Omitted
Minnesota	32	24.5	1.7	3.0
N. Dakota	32	21.3	1.4	4.6
Iowa	32	16.1	1.9	5.9

16

among these categories, particularly between omissions and substitutions, are statistically significant.

A three-by-three analysis of variance was done on the scores of the three categories—correct, substituted and omitted. The analysis showed that when the interaction value is used as the error term, the differences among the three categories are highly significant statistically. It provides evidence that the null hypothesis may be rejected at the .005 level of confidence. Although the differences among the three categories are significant, the differences among the groups of subjects from the three states on the other hand are not significant.

The final task was to test the significance of the difference between omission and substitution errors. When tests are run on the pairs of differences between the two types of errors for each of the three groups, it was found that all are statistically significant, one at the 2% level and two at the 1% level of confidence.

Since the purpose of the study was to test whether the relationship of substitution and omission errors, which was found with normal children, holds also for the pronunciation of five consonants by children having cerebral palsy, it is interesting to learn that it does not. Rather, omissions occur significantly more frequently than substitution errors for each of the three cerebral palsied groups. In this respect, the speech of children with cerebral palsy differs from that of normal children.

Chapter 4

A Second Short Test

B ECAUSE THE ADMINISTRATION of long tests is burdensome and fatiguing for children with cerebral palsy to un-
dergo, the feasibility of using a short test was investigated and
reported in Chapter 1. In that study a test was constructed involving five consonants in three positions in fifteen words. Four
criteria of test construction are the reliability of the test, its difficulty, its discriminating power and the uniqueness of its items.
It was found that the test adequately met these four criteria. The
purpose of the present study is to determine if a test composed of
six other consonants likewise will meet these four criteria.

PROCEDURE

One hundred and fifteen children with cerebral palsy, ranging
in age from 3 to 15 years, were given a test of eighteen words with
the six consonants in the initial, medial and final positions. The
children were from the states of Iowa, New York, Massachusetts
and Rhode Island. The consonants were f, v, ð, ⊖, g and k. The
word list and an alternate list is included in Chart 2 in the
appendix. Since it was found that verbal tests are somewhat
superior to picture tests, especially in the medial position, the
present research made use of only verbal items.

RESULTS

Reliability of the Test

To determine the reliability of the test, formula No. 20 by
Kuder-Richardson (1937) was used. The reliability correlations
derived by the formula are given for the items in the initial,
medial and final positions in Table 10. The reliability coefficients

18

TABLE 10
Reliability Correlations for Each of Three Verbal Subtests

Position	r
Initial	.77
Medial	.78
Final	.79

are .77 for the initial position, .78 for the medial and .79 for the final position. Pooling the scores for the three positions and using Hoyt's method (1941) of determining reliability by means of a formula based on an analysis of variance, the coefficient of reliability was .91. The standard error of measurement was .059. Thus, the reliability of this short test is quite satisfactory and comparable to that of the previous test.

Difficulty Range of the Items

The difficulties of the six consonants in the speech of those children are recorded as percentages in Table 11. The overall range is from 27% to 83%, the median being 64%. The consonant g in the initial position passed by 83% of the cases represents the easiest consonant and the consonant f in the final position, passed by only 27%, is the most difficult one. This is an acceptable range of difficulty for test items and compares favorably with the range of difficulty for the items in the previous test. It will be noticed again that the order of difficulty varies for the three positions, although the voiced continuant f is the most difficult in both the initial and medial positions. The table indicates that, on the whole, initial consonants are easiest with a mean percent of 76.3, medial consonants are the next in difficulty with

TABLE 11
Order of Difficulty of Six Consonants in Terms of Percentages

Initial		Medial		Final	
ð	70	f	54	ð	27
f	73	k	59	f	39
⊖	77	⊖	63	⊖	40
k	78	v	65	g	41
v	78	ð	67	v	43
g	83	g	74	k	61
Mean	76.3		63.7		41.8

TABLE 12
Discriminating Power of Six Consonants in Three Positions

	Initial	Medial	Final
f	.81	.86	.90
v	.75	.82	.68
ð	.83	.85	.76
⊖	.61	.80	.88
g	.78	.80	.79
k	.76	.65	.79

a mean percent of 63.7, and final consonants, with a mean percent of 41.8, are the most difficult. This order is consistent with the earlier findings.

Discriminating Power of the Items

The discriminating power or diagnostic values of an item, measured by comparing the scores of the upper 27% of the cases with those of the lower 27% can be determined by means of Flanagan's table (1939) of product moment correlations. The cofficients indicating the discriminating power of the six consonants in the three positions are given in Table 12. They range from .61 to .90. The median coefficient is .80. In a good test the discriminating power of the items should be higher than coefficients measuring the uniqueness of the items.

Uniqueness of the Items

The uniqueness of items of a test is determined by their inter-correlations and may be measured by the phi coefficient. The coefficients of the six consonantal items in each of the three positions are presented in Table 13. It is seen that they range from .19 to .57. This range is lower than that for the discriminating power. Moreover, the two ranges do not overlap. The median value for uniqueness is .39; this is much lower than the median value of .80 for the discriminating power of these items.

CONCLUSIONS

There is strong evidence that the present short test based on six consonants adequately meets the four criteria of a satisfactory testing instrument. The coefficient of reliability for this test is

TABLE 13
Phi Coefficients of Six Consonantal Items

		v	ð	⊖	*g*	*k*
	I	.19	.37	.43	.47	.49
f	M	.29	.45	.43	.37	.39
	F	.32	.20	.34	.49	.54
	I	.46	.39	.39	.23	
v	M	.33	.39	.29	.51	
	F	.34	.46	.55	.37	
	I	.39	.49	.39		
ð	M	.53	.37	.32		
	F	.39	.28	.50		
	I	.43	.41			
⊖	M	.42	.49			
	F	.20	.29			
	I	.57				
g	M	.37				
	F	.37				

.91, the standard error of measurement is .059. The range of difficulty of the items is from 27% to 83%. The discriminating power is measured by quite high product moment coefficients of correlation, and low phi coefficients indicate the uniqueness of the items. The median coefficient for the former is .80 and for the latter it is .39. Thus, on the basis of these four criteria of test construction, this short test, as was the case of a previous test, is a useful instrument with children who have cerebral palsy.

Chapter 5

Validation of Short Consonant Articulation Tests

IN THE PREVIOUS CHAPTER a short articulation test composed of six consonants for use with cerebral palsied children was described. Another short test was constructed using five consonants. These studies dealt with the determination of the reliability of the test, the range of difficulty of the items, their discriminating power and their uniqueness. There remains the further task of determining the validity of these tests. The problem of estimating the validity of a new test in an area in which a generally accepted criterion test does not exist is a very difficult one to handle with high precision. The purpose of this chapter is to present such evidence as is available for the validity of the two tests.

The conventional method for the empirical validation of a new test is to administer it together with a generally accepted standardized test to a sample of subjects and then to correlate the two sets of scores. If the correlation is reasonably high, the practice is to accept it as evidence of the validity of the new test. This is validation against a criterion.

In the field of cerebral palsied speech, there is no widely accepted standardized test with which a new instrument might be correlated, consequently at the present time there is no possibility of establishing the validity of a new consonant test for those with cerebral palsy by means of the conventional criterion technique. Therefore, it becomes necessary to seek other approaches to the problem.

One of the approaches is the extreme groups method (Anastasi, 1955; Adkins, 1947). If a test is given to two extreme groups which are selected on some other basis than the test itself, the difference between the test score means of the two groups may be taken as evidence for or against the validity of the new test. In the present studies, the children with cerebral palsy were rated by physicians and physical therapists according to the degree of gross paralytic involvement as mild, moderate and severe. Thus, it is possible to compare the consonant scores made by the mildly involved and the severely involved groups. If the null hypotheses for the differences between them is rejected, it may be accepted as evidence for the validity of the test.

The first test to be considered is composed of the six consonants; *f, v, ð, ⊖, g* and *k*. This test was in two forms both of them verbal. For this analysis, there were thirty-four mildly involved and thirty-seven severely involved children available. The mean for the mild cases was 14.0, for the severe it was 8.1. The t-score for the difference of 5.9 was 5.34. With 69 df, the probability of rejecting the null hypothesis lies at the .001 level. The significant difference of performance favoring the mildly involved group, therefore, may be taken as evidence for the validity of this test.

The alternate or second form of the test was subjected to the same kind of analysis. This form was given to the thirty-four mildly involved and thirty-seven severely involved children. The mean score for the mildly involved subjects was 14.6; for the severely involved, it was 6.7. The t-score for the difference of 7.9 is 5.87. The probability that the difference between the two groups lies at the .001 level.

In Chapter 1, a short articulation test in two forms, a verbal and a picture test composed of five consonants, was described. The consonants were *b, p, m, d* and *t*.

TABLE 14
Validity of Four Consonant Tests for Children with Cerebral Palsy
by Means of the Method of Extreme Groups

Test of Six Consonants	*Means for Mild*	*Means for Severe*	*diff*	*t*	*df*	*p*
Verbal Form 1	14.0	8.1	5.9	5.34	69	.001
Verbal Form 2	14.6	7.9	6.7	5.87	69	.001
Five Consonants						
Verbal Form	11.8	9.3	2.5	2.00	48	.05
Picture Form	11.2	8.5	2.7	2.13	49	.05

For the verbal form of the test, there were seventeen mildly involved cases and thirty-three severe ones. The mean for the former was 11.8, for the latter it was 9.3. The t-score for the difference of 2.5 was 2.00. With 48 df the probability of rejecting the null hypothesis was at the .05 level.

Table 14 summarizes these results. For the four tests, it indicates the differences between the mild and severe groups, the values and the significant levels. The differences in all four groups are in favor of the mildly involved groups.

CONCLUSION

In the absence of a criterion test with which to correlate the results of these short consonant articulation tests, the method of extreme groups has been resorted to in order to secure an estimate of the validity of these tests. With the rejection of the null hypotheses for each of the four differences between the mildly and the severely involved groups, there is an accumulation of evidence for the validity of these articulation tests for use with cerebral palsied children.

Chapter 6

A Third Short Consonant Test

THIS IS THE THIRD in a series of short consonant tests for use with children with cerebral palsy. The purpose of the present study is to determine if an instrument composed of another set of six consonants also will meet the several criteria for the standardization of a test. Among these criteria are the following: (1) the reliability of the test, (2) the difficulty of the items, (3) their discriminating power, (4) the uniqueness of the items and (5) the validity of the test.

PROCEDURE

Two hundred and twenty-six children with cerebral palsy ranging in age from 3½ to 19 years were tested with a list of seventeen words whose structure included six consonants in the initial, medial and final positions. The children were from the states of Tennessee, South Carolina, Georgia, Florida, Alabama, Louisiana and Iowa. The consonants were s, z, ʃ, ʒ, r and ļ. Since ʒ is not found in the initial position in words, it would not be included in this position in the test. (The word list is printed in Chart 3 of the Appendix.)

RESULTS

Reliability of the Test

Using Kuder-Richardson's formula (1937) for the reliability of the test, the correlations for the items in each of the initial, medial and final positions are respectively .59, .70 and .65. When the items for the three positions are pooled and applying Hoyt's formula (1941) with values derived from an analysis of variance, the coefficient of reliability is .81 and the standard error of measurement is .08.

Difficulty Range of the Items

The percentage of difficulty range of the six consonants in the articulation of these children is from 27% to 78% with a median of 61%. This range compares favorably with those of the two previous tests. Again it will be evident that the difficulty of consonants varies with their position in words.

Discriminating Power of the Items

The discriminating power of an item is measured by its correlation with the whole test. One method of calculating this relationship is by means of Flanagan's table of product moment correlations (1939). The discriminating power of each of the six consonants in the three positions with the exception of ʒ in the initial position range from .57 to .87. The median is .80.

Uniqueness of the Items

Intercorrelations as determined by the phi coefficient provide means of determining the uniqueness of the items of a test. The ʒ sound in the initial position, of course, is excepted. The range of the coefficients of intercorrelation of the six items varies from .21 to .59. There is a relationship between the discriminating power of the items of a test and their uniqueness. The principle is that the latter should be much lower than the former. The range for the discriminating power is .57 to .87, while that for the uniqueness is .21 to .59. Moreover, the median value for discriminating power is .80 while that for uniqueness is .37. In this respect the test meets the requirement of this relationship.

Validity of the Test

There remains the problem of meeting the fifth criterion of an acceptable test, namely its validity. The method of extreme group was employed in validating the present test. Two different sets of external ratings on the subjects were secured. In one the cerebral palsied children were rated by physicians or physical therapists according to the degree of gross paralytic involvement: mild, moderate and severe. The two extreme groups according to this set of ratings are the mild and severely paralyzed cases. If the difference between the means of the consonant scores of these two groups is significant statistically, then this may be accepted as evidence for the validity of the test. The difference between the means was 3.2, $t = 4.09$, $p = .001$.

A second rating was secured of the general speech ability of the children. The speech therapists rated the speech of each child as good, medium or poor. Thus again the method of extreme groups could be applied using the consonant scores of the groups whose speech was rated good and poor. This difference amounted to 8.0, $t = 15.44$, and $p = .001$. Thus on the basis of the method of extreme groups there is satisfactory evidence for the validity of the test.

CONCLUSION

It is apparent that this short test made up of a set of six consonants meets five criteria of test construction in an acceptable manner. The coefficient of reliability is .81 and the standard error of measurement is .08. The range of difficulty of the item is 27% to 87%. The median discriminating power is .80. The median phi coefficient indicating the uniqueness of the items is .37. The validity of the test as determined by the method of extreme groups using two separate external criteria is adequate. Thus it is reasonable to assume on the basis of the statistical evidence that this test should prove useful with cerebral palsied children.

Chapter 7

Correct Status of a Third Set of Consonants

I N TWO PREVIOUS STUDIES the correct status of the articulation of consonants by children with cerebral palsy was reported. The present study is an investigation of the status of articulation of another set of six consonants. The consonants are *s, z, ʃ, ʒ, r* and *l*. It will be noted that the list includes some of the most frequently defective sounds in the speech of both children and adults.

The aims of the investigation are to determine (1) the degree of observer reliability which may be attained with this set of phonemes; (2) if differences exist in the articulation of these sounds in the initial, medial and final positions in words; (3) if the degree of paralysis (mild, moderate and severe) is a factor; (4) what the relation is to the intelligence quotient; (5) what the effect of chronological age is; (6) what the effect of sex is; and (7) what the relation is to scores on the Westlake Oral Test.

PROCEDURE

The analysis was concerned with the correct articulation of the six consonants as they occurred in seventeen words. Each sound appeared in the initial, medial and final positions in the words listed in Chart 3 (see Appendix) with the exception of the consonant *ʒ* which does not appear in the initial position.

Since it had been found that a verbal test was slightly more effective than a picture test, a word test only was used with this group of subjects. The child's responses were recorded on tape and other pertinent information was also gathered. In addition to the list of words a modification of Westlake's (1951) test of oral muscular function and of respiration was administered to each child. This list is composed of items for testing control of the

28

tongue, lips and mandible. It also included items on the control of breathing.

RESULTS

Reliability of the Observer

Since this type of research project stands or falls on the accuracy with which the tape is read and the responses transcribed, observer reliability for this test was determined by independent readings of the tape by two transcribers using the responses of twenty subjects. In a total of 340 consonantal sounds, 310 were agreements and 30 were disagreements. Using the formula $\dfrac{A}{A + D}$ where A represents agreements and D disagreements the resulting reliability is 91%. This value is comparable to observer reliabilities reported earlier.

Observer reliability in the use of the oral and respiratory test was determined by independent recording by two observers using twenty-three cerebral palsied subjects. Since the means of the scores of the two observers are 62.4 and 62.5, and also since the ranges of the scores are about the same, 11 to 129, this provides evidence that the test was used with a high degree of observer reliability.

The Effect of Sex

Table 15 gives the names of correct articulation of the boys and girls in the initial, medial and final positions in words and also the means of the pooled scores. It is seen that the means for the pooled position scores are 10.15 for boys and 9.83 for girls. When these mean values are rounded they are practically the same. The variances are homogeneous. The analysis of variance indicated that no significant sex difference exists in the three positions.

TABLE 15
Means for the Sexes in Three Consonantal Positions

	N	*Total*	*Initial*	*Medial*	*Final*
Boys	132	10.15	3.47	3.88	2.80
Girls	94	9.83	3.54	3.85	2.44

TABLE 16
Means for Three Consonantal Positions

Position	Total	N	Mean
Initial	788	226	3.49
Medial	870	226	3.85
Final	597	226	2.64

The Effect of Position

Table 16 presents the means for the initial, medial and final positions of the consonants in words. It will be noted that the mean for the final position is less than for the initial and medial positions. The variances are homogeneous. This is consistent with the results of previous studies.

An analysis of variance was done using a two-factor design, the two factors being position and sex. Position differences are such that the null hypotheses may be rejected at the .001 level. In order to learn which among the three position differences are significant, t-tests were run. The difference between the consonants in the initial and medial positions is less than the critical difference and thus is not significant. In this respect the result is not consistent with that of the previous studies. It may be explained by the fact that there is one consonant less in the initial position. The consonant 3 does not occur in this position. However, the differences between the initial and final, and the medial and final, being greater than the critical difference, are statistically acceptable.

Relation to Degree of Involvement

Another problem is concerned with the speech status of cerebral palsied children in the three categories of mild, moderate and severe degrees of involvement. In the analysis of this problem these categories were further broken down into the three positions of

TABLE 17
Consonant Means by Degree of Involvement and Three Positions

Degree of Involvement	N	Initial Scores N	M	Medial Scores N	M	Final Scores N	M	Pooled Scores N	M
Mild	56	224	4.00	257	4.59	188	3.37	669	12.12
Moderate	82	306	3.73	342	4.17	239	2.91	887	10.81
Severe	88	263	2.99	274	3.11	175	1.99	712	8.09

initial, medial and final. The data are found in Table 17. It is evident that for the positions pooled the mean (right column) for the mild cases exceeds that of the moderate, while the latter exceeds that of the severely involved subjects. The difference of the means of the pooled scores for mild and moderate was found not to be significant, but the difference between the means of the pooled scores for mild and severe and for moderate and severe are significant. When the significance of the differences of the means of the mild, moderate and severe groups was determined for each of the three positions the results were tabulated in Table 18. It is apparent that the null hypothesis for mean differences between the mild and moderate for the three positions must be retained, but for the remaining differences the null hypothesis may be rejected.

Relation to the IQ

One hundred and forty-three of the children had been given mental tests. The mean IQ was 79.5, the range was 36 to 116. The mean for the correct consonant scores was 10.4, the range 1 to 17. The correlation of the consonant scores and the IQ scores was .218 ± .071. This value is significant at the 1% level but obviously it is too low for predictive purposes.

Relation to Chronological Age

The mean age of these 226 cerebral palsied children was $9\frac{1}{2}$ years, the range $3\frac{1}{2}$ to 19 years. In order to determine the strength of whatever relationship exists, a Pearson r was de-

TABLE 18
t Values for Differences of Means Between Mild, Moderate and Severe Groups in Each of Three Positions

		dif	*t*	*p*
Mild vs Moderate	Initial	.27	1.25	.20
	Medial	.42	1.22	.20
	Final	.46	1.52	.20
Mild vs Severe	Initial	1.01	0.56	.50
	Medial	1.48	4.46	.001
	Final	1.38	1.40	.001
Moderate vs Severe	Initial	.74	2.79	.01
	Medial	1.06	3.11	.01
	Final	.92	2.69	.01

termined. The correlation of age and correct scores was .181 ± .065. This correlation is significant at the 1% level but this value also is too low for predictive purpose with these consonants. That is to say, knowing the chronological age of a cerebral palsied child will not be evidence of his consonantal mastery any more than knowing his IQ will afford an accurate prediction of his speech status. This finding is consistent with those of a study of six other consonants.

Relation of Correct Articulation Scores to Oral and Respiratory Functions

Westlake (1949) has devised a test for examining the functioning of oral and respiratory function. A modification of this test will be found in Chart 17 in the Appendix. The chart includes items for scoring tongue, lip and mandible movements and also respiratory items. The oral items were scored in terms of the number of successful movements in a ten-second period. Respiratory items were scored as the number of seconds of sustained exhilation. The correlation between correct articulation scores and oral movements was .534 ± .049. The r for correct speech scores and respiration was .296 ± .063, while the r for oral and respiratory scores was .510 ± .051. The multiple correlation of speech, oral and respiratory scores was .534. The standard error of estimate was 4.07. Thus the two predictor factors of oral and breathing scores teamed together yield a correlation no higher than that between the speech and the oral factors.

SUMMARY

The analyses of the data of this study indicates that the following factors are effective in the articulation of the six consonants in the speech of children with cerebral palsy.

1. The position of the consonants in words. The null hypothesis may be rejected at the .01 level between the means of the initial and final and between the means of the medial and final positions.

2. The degree of involvement. The differences between the means of the positions pooled are significant as between

mildly and severely involved, and those between moderately involved are significant.

3. Oral function. The correlation between correct articulation scores and the muscular movements of the mouth was .534 ± .049.

The following variables were found to be ineffective or only slightly effective in the articulation of these six consonants: (1) sex, (2) chronological age, (3) IQ and (4) respiratory function. In addition, the reliability of the independent reading of tape recordings by two observers was 91% and the mean scores of oral and respiratory function by two independent observers were identical and the ranges the same.

Chapter 8

A Fourth Short Consonant Test

THIS IS THE FOURTH in a sequence of short articulation tests for evaluating the speech sound status of children with cerebral palsy. Other tests have been described previously. The present one is composed of seven consonants: w, $\textsc{m}$, j, η, η, $t\int$, $d\textit{ʒ}$. They are included in the next words. As in the previously reported instruments, an attempt was made to meet the following criteria for the standardization of a test: (1) its reliability, (2) the range of difficulty of the items composing it, (3) their discriminating power, (4) their uniqueness and (5) the validity of the test. The purpose of the present study is to determine if this test successfully meets these criteria.

1.	ring	–ŋ
2.	chair	t∫–
3.	age	–dʒ
4.	we	w–
5.	finger	–ŋ–
6.	teacher	–t∫–
7.	why	ʍ–
8.	pigeon	–dʒ–
9.	nowhere	–ʍ–
10.	you	j–
11.	not	n–
12.	onion	–j–
13.	sunny	–n–
14.	awake	–w–
15.	much	–t∫–
16.	on	–n
17.	jack	dʒ–

PROCEDURE

Two hundred twenty-three children with cerebral palsy ranging in age from 3½ to 17 years were the subjects. They were from the states of Tennessee, South Carolina, Georgia, Florida, Alabama, Louisiana and Iowa.

RESULTS

Reliability of the Test

The reliability correlations for the subtests dealing with the initial, medial and final positions of the consonants are respectively .60, .67 and .56. When the scores for the three positions are pooled and Hoyt's reliability formula (1944) is applied, the coefficient of reliability for the test as a whole is .89 with a standard error of measurement of .06. Thus the test fairly adequately meets the first of the five criteria listed above.

Difficulty Range of the Items

The percentages of difficulty of the items and the range are found in Table 19. It extends from 22% to 89%. This is an acceptable range and is comparable to those found for the other consonant tests. The orders of difficulty of the consonants in the three positions also are indicated in the table.

Discriminating Power of the Items

The discriminating power of the items of a test refers to the correlation of the scores on an item with the scores of the test as a whole. It may be calculated by means of Flanagan's table (1939). The correlations range from .53 to .90. The median is .78. It may be mentioned again that the operation which establishes the discriminating power of items also confirms their validity.

TABLE 19
Difficulty Range of Seven Consonants in Terms of Percentages

			Position		
Initial		*Medial*		*Final*	
n	89	w	83	n	73
w	87	n	76	ŋ	70
ʃ	81	ŋ	74	t ʃ	46
t ʃ	61	ʃ	63	dʒ	45
dʒ	60	t ʃ	62	*	
M	41	dʒ	59	*	
ŋ*		M	22	*	
Mean	70		63		59
Range	22% to 89%				
Median	63%				

*This sound is not present in this position.

Uniqueness of the Items

The uniqueness of the items is determined by their intercorrelations. Phi coefficients were used. The values range from .06 to .77. It will be seen that only two of them exceed .50. In general, however, the coefficients are below .50 with a median of .33 and thus are acceptable indices of the uniqueness of the items.

In a well-standardized test the correlations for the uniqueness of items should be lower than those for discriminating power. In this test the median value for the former is .33 and for the latter it is .78. Thus the test fulfills the required relationship between these two measures.

Validity of the Test

In order to present evidence for the validity of the test, the method of extreme groups was employed. In this study two sets of ratings of subjects based on different external criteria were secured. In one the cerebral palsied children were rated according to the degree of gross paralytic involvement by physicians and physical therapists. The ratings are in terms of mild, moderate and severe, the two extreme groups of course in this case are the mild and severe. A second rating was made by the speech therapist. It was based on her judgment of the general all-round speech and language ability of the child. The rating was in terms of good, medium or poor. The method of extreme groups also was applied to the therapists' ratings.

The mean for mild is 12.7, for severe it is 9.4. The difference between the means of the articulation scores of the extreme groups for the degree of involvement is significant, $N = 136$, diff $= 3.3$, $t = 4.4$, $p = .001$. The mean for good is 14.8, for poor it is 7.7. For therapists ratings $N = 163$, diff $= 7.1$, $t = 13.4$, $p = .001$. The test quite adequately meets five statistical criteria for test construction. It is reasonable to assume that this test, made up of seven consonants and standardized on 223 children from seven states, together with the three previously reported tests, may be used profitably by speech therapists for evaluating the articulation of consonant sounds of children with cerebral palsy.

The next project in this program is the restandardization of a number of other articulation tests with a view to their appropriate use with cerebral palsied children.

levels by combining the data of adjacent years. Thus the years 3 and 4 were combined into one age level, likewise years 5 and 6, and so on until the years 15 and 16. Means and standard deviations were determined for each age level. They are given in Table 20.

The table suggests that the mean age progression in the correct articulation of the blends is somewhat irregular. The apparent trend in the data was tested by a one-way analysis of variance of the scores to see if its rise from the horizontal was a significant one.

Since df = 6, F = 1.24 and p = 20%, it is obvious that the trend line does not depart significantly from the horizontal and that the chronological age factor has little effect on the articulation of these blends.

The Effect of Mental Age

The next problem to be considered is the effect of mental age on the scores. Since none of the children yielded mental ages above fourteen years, only six age levels are included. Not all the children were given mental tests. The N in this analysis is 61. Table 21 gives the results.

On inspection the means appear to exhibit a mental age progression but an analysis of variance fails to confirm this.

The Effect of Sex

The mean for fifty-one boys is 15.2 ± 6.5. For girls it is 12.7 ± 7.9. It would appear that the mean of the boys exceeds that of the girls. In order to find out if the difference between the means is statistically significant, a simple analysis of variance was run.

The difference in the means of boys and girls was not sufficient to reject the null hypotheses. It was noted above that although the

TABLE 21
Means by Mental Age Levels of Initial Double Consonant Blends

Age Levels	N	M	σ
3–4	15	16.3	6.9
5–6	10	14.6	8.0
7–8	17	18.7	4.8
9–10	8	18.1	6.3
11–12	9	17.0	5.7
13–14	2	22.5	5.0

mean for girls is less than that for boys, the standard deviation for girls exceeds that for boys. To determine if the variances of the two groups were homogeneous, a Bartlett test was made resulting in a chi square of 8.09. For 1 df the P value is .01. The variances, therefore, are heterogeneous, that for girls exceeding that for boys. Thus while the difference in means of the two sexes is negligible the girls are more variable.

Relation to Medical Diagnosis

Inasmuch as the number of athetoid children in the sample is much less than that of spastics it was considered advisable in dealing with this problem to match each athetoid with one from the spastic group. The matching was done by extent of paralytic involvement, degree of involvement, sex, age and IQ. There were sixteen matched pairs distributed as follows:

Quadriplegic Moderately Involved	5
Quadriplegic Severely Involved	10
Quad and Para Mildly Involved	1
o =	16

In one case a monoplegic was paired arbitrarily with a paraplegic, both being mildly involved. These were the only two of this degree of involvement available. The two tension athetoids were arbitrarily included in the athetoid group and were matched with spastics. Chronological ages were comparable within a year, and the IQs of each pair with one exception were within 10 points. Boys were matched with boys and girls with girls. There were seven pairs of girls and nine of boys. It will be noted that most of the pairs were moderately or severely involved. Thus the sample, although small in number, represents children whose muscular paralysis is unquestioned. The ages ranged from 4 to 15 years. Table 22 presents the results of the comparison of spastics and athetoids.

It is interesting to note that the means for spastics and athetoids

TABLE 22

Mean Scores on Initial Double Consonant Blends of Matched Spastic and Athetoid Children

	N	M	σ
Spastic	16	15.25	8.04
Athetoid	16	15.19	5.59

the observer, (2) the reliability of the test, (3) the difficulty range of the items, (4) age progression in the scores, (5) discriminating power of the items, (6) uniqueness of the items and (7) the validity of the test. The reliability of reading the responses from tape was 95%. The reliability of the test as determined by a Kuder-Richardson formula was .94. The range of difficulty of the items was found to be from 51% to 83%. The discriminating power of the items ranged from .67 to .90 with a mean of .80. The uniqueness of the items of the test ranged from .14 to .69 with a mean of .43. The validity of the test was determined by means of the method of extreme groups. The difference between the means of children rated very good and very poor on general speech and language ability amounted to 13.8 which is significant at the .001 level. In general the Templin test of initial double consonant blends appears to be suitable for use with children with cerebral palsy.

Chapter 10

Correct Status of Initial Double Consonant Blends

~~~~~~

THE ABILITY OF cerebral palsied children to use double consonant blends needs to be investigated. For this purpose the twenty-three initial double consonant blends compiled in a list by Templin (1957) was used in this study.

The aims of the investigation are concerned with (1) the effect of chronological age, (2) the effect of mental age, (3) the effect of sex, (4) the relation to the medical diagnosis of spasticity and athetosis, (5) the relation to the extent of paralytic involvement such as quadriplegia, paraplegia, and so forth, (6) the relation to the degree of involvement (mild, moderate and severe) and (7) the relation to general speech and language ability.

PROCEDURE

The study was concerned with the correct articulation of twenty-three double consonant blends as they occurred in the initial position in words. The child's verbal responses were recorded on tape.

RESULTS

The Effect of Chronological Age

In order to estimate the effect of chronological age from 3 to 16 years inclusive the fourteen years were reduced to seven age

TABLE 20
Means by Chronological Age Levels on Initial Double Consonant Blends

Age Level	N	M	σ
3–4	8	10.1	7.0
5–6	12	14.2	7.6
7–8	20	17.3	6.3
9–10	16	16.0	5.7
11–12	18	19.0	4.5
13–14	9	16.7	5.2
15–16	12	17.6	7.1

have discriminating power if its correlation with the test is relatively high. The *rs* range from .67 to .98 with a mean of .80.

The six double consonant blends which best discriminate the speech of children with cerebral palsy are in the following order: *st, sw, sk, fl, fr* and *tw.* It is interesting to note that these blends are included in the ten most difficult ones but are not in the same order.

A condition concerning the relation between discriminating power of items and their difficulty is that they must not be correlated. The value of the correlation for the twenty-three items derived by the method of rank difference is .20. Although the same ten blends head the two lists, the correlation between the complete lists is negligible.

Uniqueness of the Items

The term "uniqueness of items" means that two items should not perform the same function in a test.

In a well-standardized test a relationship exists between the discriminating power and the uniqueness of the items. The correlations for the former should be high, while those for the latter should be low. The mean *r* for discriminating power of items of this test is .80, the range being .67 to .90. The mean *r* for uniqueness is .43 and the range is .14 to .69. Thus the relationship holds for this test in a very satisfactory manner.

Validity of the Test

The validity of the test was determined by the method of extreme groups. The external criterion was a rating on the general speech and language ability of the child, his ability to communicate and his intelligibility as judged by the speech therapist in terms of very good, good, medium, poor and very poor. The mean articulation scores yielded by the test were 21.9 for those rated very good, 19.7 for those rated good, 15.4 for the medium group, 11.5 for the poor and 8.1 for the very poor.

A t-test was applied to the articulation scores of children rated on general language ability as very good and very poor. With a probability value at the .001 level for the difference in means between the two extreme groups the evidence indicates that the

Templin test of initial double consonant blends possesses quite adequate validity when used with children with cerebral palsy.

DISCUSSION

Since the purpose of the study was to standardize the Templin test of initial double consonant blends for use with cerebral palsied children, an attempt was made to see if it meets a number of criteria in the construction of a test. Of the seven analyses made of the data, five of them provide quite satisfactory results. These are the reliability of the observer, the reliability of the test, the discriminating power of the items, their uniqueness, and the validity of the test. Moreover, in an adequately constructed test there is a relationship between discriminating power and uniqueness of items. The range of the correlation coefficients of the former should be higher than those for the uniqueness of items. In this respect also this test is quite satisfactory.

The test has two weak features. The range of difficulty of the items is rather narrow. It would perhaps be preferable if it were from about 10% to 80% or 90% instead of 51% to 83%. It may be, however, that an extenuating circumstance exists with children with cerebral palsy. In previous work on consonantal articulation it also was found that consonants in the initial position are easier for these children and that the spread is not as great as with medial and final consonants.

On the whole, though, it is evident from the preceding analyses that the Templin test is suitable for evaluating the ability of children with cerebral palsy to articulate initial double consonant blends.

SUMMARY

Templin's test of initial double consonant blends was given to 103 children with cerebral palsy ranging in age from 3 to 16 years. They resided in the states of Kansas, Oklahoma, Texas, New Mexico, Arizona and California.

The aim of the study was to see if the Templin test for initial double consonant blends when standardized on cerebral palsied children can be used to evaluate the articulation of this type of child. Seven analyses of the data were made: (1) the reliability of

Chapter 9

Restandardization of the Templin Initial Double Consonant Blend Test

FOUR REPORTS on short articulation tests for evaluating the speech sound status of children with cerebral palsy were concerned with single consonants in the initial, medial and final positions in words. The present problem concerns the standardization of the Templin test (1957) of initial double consonant blends on a group of cerebral palsied children. In order to use it with cerebral palsied children, it must be restandardized on a group of these children. In standardizing the test an attempt will be made to learn if it meets the usual criteria. A general aim then of this part of the study is to find out if the Templin tests for blends are suitable for use with cerebral palsied children.

PROCEDURE

One hundred and three children with cerebral palsy ranging in age from 3 to 16 years were subjects. They were from speech clinics and rehabilitation centers in Wichita, Kansas; Norman, Oklahoma; Amarillo, Texas; Albuquerque, New Mexico; Tucson and Phoenix, Arizona; and San Diego and Santa Barbara, California. The list of double consonant blends included in the test and the key words follows.

Initial Double Consonant Blends
Templin's List

1.	pl—	pleasure	13.	fl—	flow
2.	pr—	prompt	14.	fr—	freeze
3.	tr—	train	15.	thr—	three
4.	tw—	twinkle	16.	shr—	shrink
5.	cl—	clown	17.	sk—	skate
6.	kr—	cracker	18.	sl—	sleep
7.	kw—	quilt	19.	sm—	smooth
8.	bl—	blocks	20.	sn—	snow
9.	br—	bread	21.	sp—	spoon
10.	dr—	drum	22.	st—	stairs
11.	gl—	glass	23.	sw—	sweep
12.	gr—	grass			

RESULTS

Reliability of the Observer

Tape records of the speech of thirteen cerebral palsied children were used to determine the reliability of the observer. A total number of three hundred double consonant blends were read independently from the tape by two observers. The mean percent of agreement was 95.

Reliability of the Test

The reliability of the test was determined by means of the Kuder-Richardson formula No. 20 (1937). The r value was .94. Thus this Templin test when used with children with cerebral palsy meets the criterion of test reliability quite adequately.

Difficulty Range of the Items

The difficulty of an item in a test is determined by the number of testees passing it. In this test the double blend *br* passed by 83% of the children is the easiest, while *sp* with which only 51% succeed is the most difficult item for cerebral palsied children. However, it is desirable that a test include items with a spread of difficulty. It is usually considered that the range of difficulty should vary from about 10% to 90%. The range from 51% to 83% does not meet this criterion. However, this result is characteristic. In previously reported studies consonants in the initial position also were found to be easier than those in the middle or final positions.

The ten most difficult initial double consonant blends for these children are *sp, st, sn, pl, sm, sk, thr, sw, fl,* and *tw.*

Discriminating Power of the Items

While the difficulty of an item is calculated from the number of individuals passing it, the discriminating power of an item refers to the requirement that the item should discriminate the individuals attempting it. That is to say, the subjects should make a variety of scores on the item, for if all did equally well on an item it would fail to discriminate the individuals. Discriminating power is measured by the correlation of the scores on an item with the scores of the test as a whole. An item is considered to

SUMMARY

The specific aims of the study were to determine if the differences among scores for the correct, substituted and omitted articulations were significantly different, if the articulation scores of children in the various centers belong to the same population, what the probability is that omission errors exceed substitution in the articulation of the blends. For this purpose the Templin test was given to 102 cerebral palsied children in Wichita, Kansas; Norman, Oklahoma; Amarillo, Texas; Albuquerque, New Mexico; Tucson and Phoenix, Arizona; and San Diego and Santa Barbara, California. Tape records were made of the childrens' responses to the verbal presentation of the words of the test.

The analysis yielded the following results. The mean score for articulating correctly the initial double consonant blends was 16.3, for the omission errors it was 4.41, the differences among these means was significant at the .001 level, the mean differences among the scores of the seven communities of correct articulations varied from 14.7 to 19.0, these differences were not significant and the variances were homogeneous, the mean differences among the scores of the seven communities of substitution errors varied from .03 to 2.7, the differences were not sufficient to reject the null hypothesis. The variances were heterogeneous but not severely so, the mean differences among the seven centers of omission errors were such as to sustain the null hypothesis and the variances were also heterogeneous but not severe, an analysis of the overall differences between means for substituted and omitted errors of these blends yielded the information that the null hypothesis could be rejected at the .001 level, the ten most frequent initial consonant blends for which other sounds were substituted are *pl, thr, shr, gl, cl, tw, fr, bl, cr* and *pr*, when the data were broken down into the mean differences of the two types of errors for each center five of the mean differences were significant and two were not, the ten most frequent blends omitted are *sp, st, sk, sn, sm, fl, sw, sl, tw* and *cr*.

Chapter 12

A Test of Final Double Consonant Blends

THIS STUDY IS an attempt to standardize the Templin test of final double consonant blends (1957) on a group of children with cerebral palsy and is part of a series of short articulation tests which are being constructed for use with this type of child. Templin standardized her test on normal children.

PROCEDURE

The subjects were 160 children with cerebral palsy ranging in age from 2 to 17 years. They were from speech clinics, rehabilitation centers and public schools in five New England states and six southern states.

RESULTS

Reliability of the Observer and of the Test

An analysis of the reliability of the observer in listening to blends recorded on tape was reported elsewhere. The mean percent of agreement between observers was 95. The reliability correlation for the test was calculated by means of a Kuder-Richardson formula. The r value was .85.

Validity of the Test

The validity of a test is determined in terms of an external criterion. Two external criteria were used in this study based on the method of extreme groups. One is the medical diagnosis of mild, moderate and severe involvement. The mean of the mild cases was 13.4 ± 4.2 and of the severe it was 11.3 ± 4.6. The difference of 2.1 was evaluated by a t-test. With df $= 101$, t $= 2.25$ the probability value was .05 in favor of the mild cases. The second external criterion consisted of ratings on a five-point scale

TABLE 24

Mean Scores of Correct, Submitted and Omitted
Initial Double Consonant Blends

		Correct		*Substituted*		*Omitted*	
	N	M	σ	M	σ	M	σ
Wichita	14	15.1	6.2	2.7	2.4	5.2	4.7
Norman	7	19.0	7.0	1.1	1.6	2.9	5.1
Amarillo	7	17.8	3.8	0.3	0.5	4.7	3.6
Albuquerque	26	15.7	6.7	2.1	2.2	5.1	5.2
Arizona	13	16.5	8.7	1.4	2.7	4.6	6.5
San Diego	17	17.0	6.8	2.3	3.4	3.3	3.9
Santa Barbara	19	14.7	7.2	2.7	2.4	4.0	3.7

articulation of the blends greatly exceeds those of both substitutions and omissions. The first problem, then, is to determine if the null hypothesis of the differences of the means of correct, substituted and omitted scores applies. The overall* mean of the correct scores is 16.3, of the substitutions it is 2.09, and of omission it is 4.41. An analysis of variance using a treatment by subjects design was applied to the data.

It was found that the differences in means among the correct, substituted and omitted blends are highly significant and that the null hypothesis may be rejected at the .001 level of confidence.

The next problem is to determine if for each of the correct, substituted and omitted groups of blends the means of the seven centers are alike and if the groups belong to the same population. For this purpose a simple analysis of variance and a Bartlett test of homogeneity of variance were performed on each of the three types of scores. The Bartlett test showed that the variances in each group were heterogeneous. The analysis of variance showed that for each group the differences among the means were not significant.

The next problem to be considered is the hypothesis that omissions of the twenty-three initial double consonant blends exceed substitutions.

The p value of .001 for the difference of 2.32 and t = 5.09 between the means of substituted and omitted errors indicates that for the sample as a whole the null hypothesis may be rejected. The omission errors exceed the substitution errors.

---

*The term "overall" as used here refers to the 102 subjects taken as a single group.

TABLE 25
Rank Order of Errors

	Substitutions			Omissions	
Blends	*Frequency*	*%*	*Blends*	*Frequency*	*%*
1. pl-	29	28.4	sp-	45	44.1
2. thr-	23	22.7	st-	39	38.2
3. shr-	21	20.5	sk-	33	32.2
4. gl-	14	13.7	sm-	32	31.3
5. cl-	14	13.7	sm-	27	26.4
6. tw-	12	11.7	fl-	23	22.5
7. fr-	12	11.7	sw-	22	21.5
8. bl-	9	8.8	sl-	20	19.6
9. cr-	9	8.8	tw-	19	18.6
10. pr-	9	8.8	cr-	17	16.6
11. fl-	8	7.8	bl-	17	16.6
12. sn-	7	6.9	tr-	16	15.7
13. sw-	6	5.9	kw-	14	13.7
14. sm-	6	5.9	gl-	14	13.7
15. sl-	6	5.9	br-	13	12.7
16. br-	6	5.9	dr-	13	12.7
17. tr-	6	5.9	gr-	13	12.7
18. kw-	5	2.9	fr-	13	12.7
19. dr-	4	3.9	pr-	11	10.7
20. gr-	4	3.9	cl-	10	9.8
21. st-	3	2.9	pl-	10	9.8
22. sk-	2	1.9	thr-	8	7.8
23. sp-	2	1.9	skr-	8	7.8

A final aim of the study was to calculate the frequencies and rank order of substitution and omission errors. Table 25 gives the results.

The table may be read: 29 or 28.4% of 102 cerebral palsied children substituted another sound for the consonant blend *pl;* and 45 or 44.1% of them omitted the blend *sp.* Note that the percent columns add up to more than 100% because many of the children made two or more substitution or omission errors. The ten initial double consonant blends most frequently substituted by other sounds by these children are *pl, thr, skr, gl, cl, tw, fr, bl, cr,* and *pr.* The ten most frequently omitted initial double consonant blends are *sp, st, sk, sn, sm, fl, sw, sl, tw* and *er.* It is seen that of the ten omitted blends, seven of them include the phoneme *s.* Only one blend, *er,* is common to both lists.

records, the effect of chronological age on the correct articulation by cerebral palsied children of the initial double consonant blends, the effect of mental age, the effect of sex, the relation to the medical diagnosis, the relation to the extent of paralytic involvement, the relation to the degree of involvement and the relation to general language ratings.

The following represent the findings of the investigation. (1) The mean percent of observer reliability was 95. The range was from 79% to 100%. (2) The mean correct scores from the chronological age level, 3 to 4 years of age to 15 to 16 years of age varied irregularly from 10.1 to 16.6. Chronological age progression was not significantly present in the scores. (3) The means for mental age from 3 to 4 years of age to 13 to 14 years of age showed no age progression in the scores. Mean sex differences in the correct articulation of the blends were not present, but girls showed significantly greater variability in articulation than boys. (5) An analysis of the scores by sixteen spastics matched for age, sex, extent of involvement and IQ with sixteen athetoids revealed that the mean scores were identical and the variances homogeneous indicating no significant statistical differences between the two groups as far as initial double consonant blends are concerned. (6) The mean differences among quadriplegics, paraplegics and hemiplegics were significant and the variances were homogeneous indicating that significant differences exist in the three groups. (7) Differences among mildly involved, moderately and severely involved cases in this sample were not statistically significant. The variances were homogeneous. (8) When the children were rated on general speech and language ability on a three-point scale as good, medium and poor, the mean differences were significant at the .001 level, and the variances were homogeneous.

Chapter 11

Substitutions and Omissions of
Initial Double Consonant Blends

IT HAS BEEN OBSERVED that substitution errors occurred more frequently than omission errors in the articulation of speech sounds by normal preschool children. A similar situation was found with children in grade one through grade six. Earlier the reverse situation was reported in the articulation of consonants by children with cerebral palsy. The purpose of the present study was to discover if the reverse situation obtains also for the articulation of initial double consonant blends by these children. Another was to determine if the scores of the children from seven communities belong to a common population. A final aim was to calculate the frequencies of substitutions and omission and to determine the ten most frequent double consonant blends in each category.

PROCEDURE

There were 102 children with cerebral palsy ranging in chronological age from 3 to 16 years. The test used with these children was the Templin Initial Double Consonant Blend Test (1957). Tape recordings were made of the children's responses and the reliability of the reading of the tape by two observers has been reported elsewhere. The term "substitution" refers to the articulation of a phoneme in place of another. The term "omission" is here defined as the dropping out of either the first or the second, or both phonemes, in the blend.

RESULTS

Table 24 gives the means of three types of scores for each of the seven groups of children.

An inspection of the table reveals that the means for correct are practically identical, but it remains to be seen if the variances are homogeneous. Accordingly, a Bartlett test was done on the data. The resulting chi-square value yielded a p of .50, the variances thus being homogeneous. Since the mean differences in articulation are nil and the variances are homogeneous, the results may be taken as evidence that as far as initial double consonant blends are concerned, spastics and athetoids belong to a common population.

Relation to Extent of Involvement

The distribution of the children according to extent of involvement indicates that fifty-eight of them are quadriplegic. Of these fifty-five are available for the analysis. There are thirteen paraplegics and eighteen hemiplegics. The numbers in the remaining categories—rigid, flaccid, ataxic, and so forth—are too few to be included. In Table 23 is found the means of the three groups.

It will be noted that the mean for the hemiplegics exceeds that of the paraplegics, and the latter is greater than the mean of the quadriplegics. Also the standard deviation of the hemiplegics is less than for the other two categories. The data on which the above means were based were subjected to an analysis of variance.

With an F ratio of 3.72 and 2 and 83 df, the probability that the differences in means among the quadriplegics, the paraplegics and the hemiplegics lies between the 5% and 2½% level.

In order to determine between which groups the differences are significant, t-tests were performed. The difference between the quadriplegics and the hemiplegics the probabilities lie at the 1% level and are therefore significant. Bartlett's test was applied to the variances which turned out to be homogeneous. Since this was the case, such differences among the three groups are due to the means and not to the variances. Thus the hemiplegics in this

TABLE 23
Extent of Involvement
Initial Double Consonant Blends

	N	M	σ
Quadriplegic	55	14.4	7.00
Paraplegic	13	16.7	6.97
Hemiplegic	18	19.3	5.06

sample do better than the other two groups. The result also may be taken as a verification of the validity of this test.

Relation to Degree of Involvement

Available for an analysis of the effect of degree of involvement upon the blend articulation of the children were thirty who were mild cases, thirty-five moderates and thirty-one severely involved subjects.

The mean of the mild cases is 16.6 ± 6.9. For the moderates it is 17.0 ± 6.5 and for the severe cases it is 14.4 ± 6.9.

The differences among the three groups were not significant and since the variances are homogeneous, the inference may be drawn that degree of involvement has little effect on the articulation of these blends.

Relation to General Speech and Language Ratings

Each cerebral palsied child was rated by his speech therapist on his general speech and language ability in terms of good, medium and poor.

The mean articulation scores of children rated on general language facility varies from 19.7 ± 4.7 for those rated good, to 15.4 ± 5.5 for the medium and 11.5 ± 6.1 for those rated poor. An analysis of variance revealed that the F value lay beyond the .001 level.

There remains the problem of the homogeneity of the variances. When Bartlett's test was applied, the chi-square value with 2 df yielded a probability value of 10%. Since the variances are homogeneous, it is the means which determine the differences.

SUMMARY

An attempt was made in this study to describe and analyze the correct status of initial double consonant blends in the speech of 102 children with cerebral palsy from 3 to 16 years of age. The list of blends is one compiled by Templin and included twenty-three items. The children were from the states of Kansas, Oklahoma, Texas, New Mexico, Arizona and California. The specific aims of the study were to investigate the degree of observer reliability which may be attained in reading the blends from tape

The difference in variability is significant at the .005 level. Since the variances are heterogeneous a modified *t* was applied to the difference between the means. The observed value of *t* was 1.885. The Cochran-Cox (1953) modified t.05 was 2.142. Since the latter is greater than the former the difference between the means of the two groups is not significant. Such difference as exists is one of the variability rather than of central tendency.

Since the left cerebral hemisphere is considered to contain the speech centers, it is remarkable to find that articulation of right and left hemiplegics is the same.

Relation to Extent of Involvement

In this sample there were available for this analysis eighty-two quadriplegics, twenty-one paraplegics and thirty-two hemiplegics. The mean of the first group was 10.9 ± 2.8.

As in the case of initial double consonant blends the mean of the quadriplegics is lower than those for hemiplegics and paraplegics. The Bartlett test applied to the variances showed them to be heterogeneous. Accordingly modified t-tests were applied to the means of the three groups. The difference between the means of the quadriplegics and the paraplegics was significant at the .01 level. However, the difference between the means of the quadriplegics and the hemiplegics was not significant, nor was the difference between the hemiplegics and paraplegics significant.

Relation to Degree of Involvement

Available for an analysis of the effect of involvement upon the articulation of the final double consonant blends were thirty-five mild cases, forty-nine moderates and sixty-eight severely involved children, a total of 152.

The mean of the mild cases was 13.4 ± 4.3 and of the moderate was 12.8 ± 4.6. For the severe it was 11.3 ± 4.3. The variance of the three groups, it will be noted is about the same. To determine if there are significant differences among the means, an analysis of variance was done. It showed that the differences among the means of scores of mildly, moderately and severely involved children is significant at the .05 level. This result is somewhat different than with initial double consonant blends for which the F ratio is not significant. It remains to learn which of these means is the determining factor. Accordingly t-tests were applied to them. The difference between the means of the mild and severely involved cases is significant at the .05 level, but those between the mild and moderate and the moderate and severe are not significant.

Distribution of IQS

A further matter concerns the proportion of these children whose mental status falls below an IQ of 90. It was found that 75% of the children in the present study had IQs of less than 90, while 72% of those who were included in the study on initial consonant blends had IQs below 90. The IQs of about 20% of the children of the present and 18% of those in the former study group fell in the normal range, 91 to 110, while the equivalent figures for those above 111 were about 5% and 10%. It may be pertinent here to report that in a third group of the cerebral palsied children the IQs below 90 averaged slightly above 70%.

SUMMARY

In this study an attempt was undertaken to analyze the correct status of final double consonant blends in the speech of 160 children with cerebral palsy from 2 to 17 years of age. The blends were those of a list of eighteen items compiled by Templin. The subjects were from the states of Maine, New Hampshire, Vermont, Massachusetts, Connecticut, Florida, Alabama, Mississippi, Louisiana, Texas and Arkansas. The aims of the study were to investigate the following factors in their effect on articulation of final blends: sex differences, age differences, the relation of spasticity and athetosis, the effect of right and left hemiplegia, the relation to extent of involvement and the relation of degree of involvement.

The results of the investigation are listed as follows. The mean percent of observer reliability was 95. Mean sex differences were not found, but the variability of the girls was greater than that of the boys. Both chronological and mental age had little

Chapter 13

Correct Status of Final Double Consonant Blends

I N THIS CHAPTER the ability of children with cerebral palsy to articulate final double consonant blends is considered. The status of the initial double consonant blends was previously reported. In the present study eighteen final double blends compiled in a list by Templin (1957) were used.

The aims of the study are to determine (1) the reliability of the reader in transcribing sounds from the tape recordings, (2) the effect of age, (3) the relation to the medical diagnosis, (4) to compare the articulatory ability of right and left hemiplegics, (5) to determine the relation of the extent of paralytic involvement and (6) the relation to the degree of involvement.

PROCEDURE

A verbal test previously had been found to be slightly more effective with these children than a picture test. Accordingly only a verbal test was used. The list of words was read to the child and he was instructed to repeat each word as it was pronounced. The responses were recorded on tape.

RESULTS

Reliability of the Observer

The ability of the observer to listen to sounds recorded on tape has been reported in a previous section. In general the agreements of two independent listeners amounts to 90%. Thus the observer error is about 10%. In the case of double consonant blends the reliability of the observer was 95%.

There is little difference between the means of boys and girls, but the girls are twice as variable as boys. This difference is significant at the .001 level. Thus such differences as exist between the sexes are due to the greater variability of the girls than to the means. A similar situation was found to exist in regard to initial double consonant blends.

Relation to Medical Diagnosis

This analysis has been restricted to a comparison of two medical categories, the phonation of final blends of spastics and athetoids. Since there are in the sample fewer athetoids than spastics, each athetoid was matched with one of the spastics in terms of sex, age, and extent and degree of paralytic involvement. There were twenty-six pairs in the sample which could be matched on this basis. It is difficult to pair exactly according to all of the four criteria, but it was possible to do so according to three of them. Ages were matched within a year with three exceptions.

The mean for the spastics was 12.3 ± 4.1. For the athetoids it was 11.2 ± 4.4. The variances were homogeneous. When a t-test was run on the difference between the means of the spastics and athetoids the probability value was at the .45 level, indicating that there is little evidence for any difference. Since the difference between the means is not significant and since the variances are homogeneous, the inference is that the mastery of blends by spastics and by athetoids is quite similar. This result was found also with initial double consonant blends.

Relation to Right and Left Hemiplegia

In order to learn if there is a difference in the phonation of final double consonant blends between right and left hemiplegics, the means and variance of the two groups were compared. There were sixteen right and fifteen left hemiplegics. The next table gives the pertinent information.

The difference between the means is 2.0, and the variance of the scores of left hemiplegics is about four times that of the right.

TABLE 27
**Mean and Variances of Scores of Final Double Consonant Blends
of Right and Left Hemiplegics**

	N	M	σ
Right	16	14.3	6.0
Left	15	12.3	25.4

present. Since the F ratio was less than 1, no trend in the scores with chronological age is discernable. This result is similar to that of the initial double consonant blends.

In the case of mental age progression, adjacent years likewise were combined. The first mental age level includes the second and third years, the second includes the fourth and fifth years and so on. There were ninety-eight cases in this sample to whom mental tests were administered.

The means for the mental age levels increase from 11.8 ± 4.6 to 15.7 ± 2.9. In order to learn if this apparent increase is statistically significant an analysis of variance was performed. The apparent trend with mental age in the scores falls short of significance at the 5% level. An absence of a significant trend was also found for initial double consonant blends.

It may be inferred, then, that there is little evidence for a significant progression in scores with respect to either chronological or mental age.

SUMMARY

Templin's test of final double consonant blends was administered to 160 children with cerebral palsy ranging in age from 2 to 17 years. They resided in the states of Maine, New Hampshire, Vermont, Massachusetts, Connecticut, New Jersey, Florida, Alabama, Mississippi, Louisiana, Texas and Arkansas.

The purpose of the study was to restandardize the Templin test of final double consonant blends for use with children with cerebral palsy.

Seven criteria were employed in the analysis: (1) the reliability of the observer, (2) the reliability of the test, (3) the validity of the test, (4) difficulty of the items, (5) their discriminating power, (6) their uniqueness and (7) chronological and mental age progression in the scores. All criteria except age progression were met. Agreement of two observers was 95%; a Kuder-Richardson formula yielded test reliability of .85; the difficulty of the items ranged from 18% to 92%; the validity of the test was determined by means of the method of extreme groups. The difference between the mean articulation scores of children rated mild and those rated severe by the medical examiner was significant at the .05 level.

The difference between the mean scores of those rated very good and those rated very poor on general language ability was significant at the .001 level; the mean r for discriminating power was .67; the range was from 149 to .87; the mean r for the uniqueness of items was .32, the range was from .04 to .68; chronological and mental age progressions in the articulation scores were not present. The Templin test of final double consonant blends, like the test on initial double consonant blends, appears to be quite adequate for use with children with cerebral palsy.

by the speech therapist of the general language ability of the child, his ability to communicate and his intelligibility. The five categories of the scale are very good, good, medium, poor and very poor. The mean score of cases rated very good was 15.8 ± 2.2. Of the very poor it was 7.2 ± 4.7. The difference was 8.6, $t = 7.54$, $df = 48$, and $p = .001$. These analyses provide evidence of the validity of the test.

Difficulty Range of the Items

The eighteen items of this test were administered to 160 subjects. In order to evaluate the difficulty of an item the number of children who passed it was determined and converted into a percent. The item passed by the largest percentage is considered to be the easiest one in the test. Conversely the smallest percent of the cases passing an item indicates that it is the most difficult. Thus the blend *kl* with a percentage of 92 is the easiest, while the blend *sp* with a percentage of 18 is the most difficult item. On the assumption that a good test is one which all the subjects will neither pass nor fail all the items, it is customary to consider that the percentage range of item difficulty should extend from about 10 to 90. In this test the item difficulty ranges from 18% to 92%. This is a much more satisfactory spread than that for initial double consonant blends reported in a previous section where the range was from 51% to 83%. The data are found in Table 26.

The ten most difficult final consonant blends are *sp, sk, st, tr, shr, fr, fl, sl, sm* and *pl*. It is interesting to note that six of these

TABLE 26
Percentage Difficulty Range of 18 Final Double Consonant Blends in the Speech of 160 Children with Cerebral Palsy

	Blend	%		Blend	%
1.	kl	92	10.	sm	79
2.	bl	92	11.	sl	78
3.	gl	89	12.	fl	76
4.	br	87	13.	fr	75
5.	kr	87	14.	shr	68
6.	gr	85	15.	tr	48
7.	pr	81	16.	st	42
8.	dr	81	17.	sk	38
9.	pl	80	18.	sp	18

final blends are also found among the initial double consonant blends, which are *sp, sk, fl, sm* and *pl.*

Discriminating Power of the Items

The discriminating power of an item means that the subjects taking the item should make a range of scores. The item should discriminate among the individuals. The discriminating power of an item is measured by the correlation of its scores with the scores of the test as a whole. If the correlation is relatively high the item is considered to be satisfactory and may be included in the test. The correlations are relatively high, ranging from r = .49 to .87 with a mean of .67.

Uniqueness of the Items

In order to determine that the items of the test do not duplicate the same function to any great degree, intercorrelations among them were calculated by means of the phi coefficient. The mean phi coefficient is .32, the range is from .04 to .68. These values should be lower than those for discriminating power. The mean *r* for the discriminating power of the items of this test is .67 which is double the phi coefficient. The range is from .49 to .87 which in general is a higher range of values than that for the phi coefficient. Thus the relationship between discriminating power and the uniqueness of items is satisfactorily met in this test.

This test in terms of item analysis of difficulty, discriminating power and uniqueness is acceptable.

Age Progression in the Scores

Age progression is reported for both chronological and mental ages. In the analysis adjacent chronological ages were combined into age levels. Thus the first level includes the second and third years, the second level includes the fourth and fifth years, and so on to the seventh which includes the fourteenth to the seventeenth years. A total of 149 cases were available for the analysis. The range of means was from 10.6 to 12.3.

A simple analysis of variance was done to see if a trend was external criteria were used, the medical diagnosis of the children and ratings by the therapist of their general language ability and communicability. The medical diagnosis was in terms of mild and severe involvement. The language ratings were in the two extremes of good and poor. The mean of the mild sample was 20.6 ± 7.4. The severe was 16.5 ± 7.4. The difference between the means of the articulation scores of children mildly and severely involved was subjected to a t-test and was found to be significant. The same procedure was followed with the means of scores of children rated good and poor in general language facility by the therapist. The mean of the group rated good was 22.1 ± 5.9 while the mean of the group rated poor was 12.4 ± 6.5.

The variances for each comparison are homogeneous. The t value of the difference between the means of children diagnosed by the physician as mild and severe is significant at the .02 level. The t value of the difference between the means of children rated good and poor by the speech therapist was significant at the .001 level. These values may be accepted as evidence for the validity of the test.

Difficulty Range of the Items

The difficulties of the items of the blend test for the 129 children are listed in order from the most to the least difficult in Table 30.

TABLE 30
**Difficulties of Final Reversed Blends in the Speech of Children
with Cerebral Palsy**

Blend	%	Blend	%	Blend	%
tl	39	rp	57	lp	66
ft	39	rd	57	th	67
lz	40	mp	57	ngk	68
nd	40	lt	58	rf	69
pt	42	rk	58	lf	72
kt	42	thr	60	rn	78
nt	48	ks	62	rm	80
rt	51	lk	62	sm	83
lb	52	rth	64	mr	88
rb	56	rg	66	nr	89

Mean: 60%
Range: 39% to 89%

The range of difficulty of these blends extends from 39% for the blend *tl* as in "bottle" to 89% for *nr* as in "thinner." The mean is 60%. Thus the distribution of the difficulty scores of the blends is skewed.

Discriminating Power of the Items

The discriminating power of a blend is measured by comparing the scores of the upper and lower 27% of the subjects. If the coefficients of correlation in general are substantial the items are assumed to discriminate the testees quite well. The *rs* range from .49 to .85 with a mean of .69.

Uniqueness of the Items

Uniqueness refers to the nonduplication of function among items of a test. If two blends correlate highly, presumably they are performing the same function. The test of the uniqueness of items of a test is that the intercorrelations must be low. The range of these intercorrelations is from .03 to .54. The mean is .27.

SUMMARY

Of the six criteria used for the standardization of the test of final double reversed consonant blends five of them are adequately met. These are test reliability, discriminating power of the items, their uniqueness and the relationship between the last two criteria. However, the distribution of the difficulties of the items is skewed. On the whole the test appears to be adequate for use with cerebral palsied children.

England cases was significantly in favor of substitutions, but that for the southern group was not significant. The most frequent substitution among final double consonant blends was *tr*. The three most frequent omissions among these blends were *sp, st* and *sk*. Comparisons between errors in initial double consonant blends and final double blends were made.

Chapter 15

Standardization of a Test of Final Double Reversed Consonant Blends

THIS CHAPTER IS another study in a series of short tests for use with children who have cerebral palsy. Templin (1957) standardized one of her final reversed consonant blend tests on 3- to 5-year-old normal children. It is necessary, however, that when a test is to be used with a particular population it first should be standardized on a sample of that population. This investigation therefore is an attempt to standardize the Templin test on a sample of children with cerebral palsy. A previous study reported the standardization of a test of initial consonant blends. An example of an item of that list is the sound *bl* as in "black." In the present study the sounds in the final blend are reversed as *lb* in "bulb."

PROCEDURE

Articulation data were collected on tape on 129 children with cerebral palsy between the ages of 3 to 16 years in the East, the South, and the Midwest.

An analysis of the data was made to learn if the test would meet six criteria for the standardization of the test: (1) the reliability of the test, (2) its validity, (3) the range of difficulty of the items, (4) the discriminating power of the items, (5) their uniqueness and (6) the relation between discriminating power and uniqueness.

RESULTS

Reliability of the Test

The reliability of the test was determined by means of the Kuder-Richardson formula No. 20. The coefficient of reliability was .89.

Validity of the Test

The method of extreme groups was applied to the data. Two

RESULTS

Table 28 gives the means and standard deviations of correct, substitution and omission scores of the two groups.

An analysis of variance and t-tests were run on the first two rows of the table. The analysis of variance showed that interaction is significant (p = .001), the differences between the means of the New England and southern groups are not significant, and the differences among the means of correct, substituted and omitted final double consonant blends are highly significant (p = .005).

Having established evidence that regional differences are not significant and recognizing from Table 28 that mean scores for correct articulation greatly exceed those for substitutions and omissions, it remains to learn if the differences between the means of the combined substitutions and combined omissions is significant. It may be noted in the third row of Table 28 that the differences amount to only 0.2 which is negligible.

It was noted that the interaction turned out to be highly significant, suggesting that the difference for the New England group may be in the opposite direction from the southern groups. Accordingly separate t-tests were applied to the differences between the two types of errors.

The small difference between the means of the two types of errors for the southern group is not significant. However, for the New England group the greater mean of the substitutions was significant at the .05 level. This is an opposite finding to that of initial double blends where omissions were more frequent. The evidence, then, is inconclusive as to the relation between substitutions and omissions in the speech of these children as far as final double blends are concerned.

Another aim of the study was to determine the rank order of substitution and omission errors. The data are given in Table 29.

The error orders of the substitutions and the omissions are not the same. The final consonant blend which is most frequently substituted is *tr* with a percentage of 18. The three final double blends most frequently omitted are *sp* with 29%, *st* and *sk* each with 23%. Presumably these are the final blends in the speech

TABLE 29
Rank Order of Substitution and Omission Errors of Final Double Consonant Blends

	Substitutions			Omissions	
Blends	Frequency	%	Blends	Frequency	%
1. tr	71	18	sp	101	30
2. fr	32	9	st	79	23
3. shr	32	9	sk	78	23
4. dr	29	8	shr	11	3
5. pl	29	8	tr	8	2
6. fl	26	6	sm	7	2
7. sl	25	6	fr	7	2
8. sm	24	6	fl	7	2
9. br	22	5	gr	7	2
10. pr	21	5	kr	6	2
11. gr	17	4	pr	6	2
12. sp	15	4	sl	5	2
13. kr	14	3	gl	4	1
14. kl	10	2	br	3	1
15. sk	10	2	bl	3	1
16. bl	9	2	kl	3	1
17. gl	7	2	pl	3	1
18. st	4				

of children with cerebral palsy with which the speech therapist might be mostly interested.

SUMMARY

The purpose of the present investigation was to determine if the articulation scores of children with cerebral palsy in New England and the Deep South belong to the same population of scores, if differences among the means of correct, substituted and omitted scores were significantly different, if there is a difference between the frequency of substitutions and omissions, and to identify the blends with which the speech therapist may find it most necessary to work.

The following results of the investigation are listed: The mean score of all cases for correctly articulating the final double consonant blends was 12.5, for substitutions it was 2.5, and for omissions is was 2.3. The differences among the means was significant at the .005 level. The difference between the means for substitutions and for omissions for all cases was negligible. The differences between the means of these errors for the New effect on the means of the scores. An analysis of the scores of twenty-six pairs of spastics and athetoids matched for age, sex, extent and degree of involvement showed no significant difference between the means or between the variance in the articulation of these blends. The mean difference between the right and left hemiplegics was not significant but the variance in the articulation of these blends by left hemiplegics was about four times that of right hemiplegics. The difference between the means of the quadriplegics and the paraplegics was such that the null hypothesis could be rejected, but the difference btween the means of the quadriplegics and the hemiplegics as well as that between the hemiplegics and paraplegics was not significant. The variances were heterogeneous. Concerning the effect of degree of involvement, the mean of the mild cases was statistically greater than that of the severe cases, but those between the mild and moderate and the moderate and severe are not significant. The variances were homogeneous. It was found that 75% of the children with cerebral palsy who served as subjects in the investigation had IQs below 90; 20% were in the normal range; and 5% had IQs above 111. Comparisons were made regarding similarities and differences in the articulation of initial and of final double consonant blends by children with cerebral palsy.

Chapter 14

Substitutions and Omissions of
Final Double Consonant Blends

IN AN INVESTIGATION of the articulation of initial double consonant blends in the speech of children with cerebral palsy, it was found that omission errors exceeded substitutions. An aim of the present study was to find out if a similar situation holds for final double consonant blends. A second purpose was to determine if the scores of children from two regions belong to a common population. A further aim was to calculate the frequencies of substitutions and omissions and to determine the most frequent final double consonant errors in each category.

PROCEDURE

included were 136 children with cerebral palsy ranging in age from 2 to 17 years in two regions, New England and the Deep South. The states of Maine, New Hampshire, Vermont, Massachusetts and Connecticut comprise one group. The southern area included Florida, Alabama, Mississippi and Louisiana. There were ninety-two subjects from the South and forty-four from New England. Templin's list of double consonant blends was administered to the children. Tape recordings were made of the verbal responses of the children.

TABLE 28

**Means and Standard Deviations of Correct, Substitution and Omission Scores
of Final Double Consonant Blends**

		Correct		Substitutions		Omissions	
	N	M	σ	M	σ	M	σ
New England	44	12.7	4.5	3.0	3.2	1.9	1.5
South	92	12.5	4.3	2.3	2.4	2.5	1.8
Combined	136	12.5	4.3	2.5	2.7	2.3	1.1

Status of Articulation of Final Reversed Consonant Blends

THE STATUS OF articulation of thirty final double reversed consonant blends by children with cerebral palsy will be dealt with in this chapter. The blends are those included in a list published by Templin.

The purposes of the investigation are to determine (1) the effect of geographical regions, (2) the effect of sex, (3) the relation of scores to chronological age, mental age and IQ of the children, (4) the relation to the medical diagnosis, (5) the relation to the extent of involvement, (6) the relation to right and left hemiplegia and (7) the frequency of correct, substituted and omitted responses.

PROCEDURES

Articulation data were secured by means of a test of final double reversed consonant blends administered to 273 children from five northeastern states, ten northern central states, nine southern states and six western states.

RESULTS

Comparison of Geographical Regions

The articulation data were classified according to four geographical regions—the eastern, northern central, southern and western states. The means and standard deviations of the scores for each region are given in Table 31.

TABLE 31

Means and Standard Deviations of Regional Scores of Final Reversed Consonant Blends

Regions	N	M	σ
Eastern	35	20.0	6.4
North Central	59	19.9	7.4
Southern	118	19.4	7.7
Western	61	21.1	6.8

In order to determine if there are regional differences among the means of Table 31 an analysis of variance was done. The Bartlett test of homogeneity of variance was applied to the data. Chi square was 5.98. With df = 3, the *p* value was found to be between .20 and .30. The variances thus are homogeneous. Since the F ratio is less than 1, and the variances are homogeneous, it is evident that regional differences in the articulation of these blends are not present. This is evidence for the reliability of this test.

The Effect of Sex

The mean for boys is 20.4, for girls 21.0 Standard deviations are 6.1 and 5.5. The difference is .06, a value too small to be significant. The absence of sex difference in the articulation of these blends is consistent with similar findings in articulation of other consonant sounds by this type of child.

Relation to Chronological Age, Mental Age and IQ

The correlation with chronological age is .31, with mental age it is .25, with IQ it is .49. An interesting matter concerning these blends is that the coefficients of correlation for this test are somewhat higher than those previously reported. In this respect these blends are exceptional.

Distribution of IQs

Of the 273 children there were 102 whose IQs were available. They were distributed as follows:

	Frequency	%
Below 40	3	3
41 – 70	40	39
71 – 90	33	33
91 –110	22	22
111 +	3	3

Twenty-two percent of the children fell in the normal mental range, 3% were above normal, 75% were below IQ 90, and 42% were below IQ 70. These values are comparable to percentages found in previous studies.

Relation to the Medical Diagnosis

A calculation was made to determine if the difference in mean articulation of the final reversed blends of spastic and athetoids was significant. Available records for this purpose were those of eighty-one spastics and twenty-four athetoids. The mean for both spastics and athetoids is 19.5. The standard deviation of the former is 7.5. For the latter it is 16.6. The standard deviation of the athetoids greatly exceeds that of the spastics. The variances thus are heterogeneous. The Cochran-Cox modified t-formula, therefore, was applied to the data resulting in $t.05 = 2.05$. Since this value far exceeds the observed t of .84, the differences between the two means is not significant. Thus with this type of blend there is no difference between the means of the spastics and athetoids but the latter are more variable.

Relation to Extent of Involvement

A comparison of the means of quadriplegics, hemiplegics and paraplegics suggests that paraplegics are superior to the other two groups. The mean of the quadriplegics is 16.8 ± 7.8. The mean of the hemiplegics is 20.0 ± 5.1, while that of the paraplegics is 21.0 ± 7.6.

In order to determine if the difference among the means of the groups are significant t-tests were applied. The difference between the means of quadriplegics and paraplegics is significant at the .05 level. This is the usual finding in this series of short tests.

Relation to Right and Left Hemiplegia

The means and standard deviations of right and left hemiplegics were determined and a t-test was applied.

The difference between the means of right and left hemiplegics is not significant. The mean of right hemiplegics was 20.4 ± 5.7. For left hemiplegics it was 19.4 ± 5.3. This is consistent with the findings in other sections of this investigation.

Correct and Incorrect Responses

An analysis was made of correct responses, omissions and substitutions. An omission of a final blend means that one or both parts of the blend is not articulated. A substitution refers to the replacement of one or both parts of the blend by another consonant or blend. The pertinent data are given next.

Without performing a statistical analysis, it is evident by in-

TABLE 32

Means and Standard Deviations of Correct Scores, Substitutions and Omissions of Final Reversed Consonant Blends

	N	M	σ
Correct	273	19.9	6.5
Substitutions	273	1.3	1.9
Omissions	273	7.9	5.8

spection that correct articulation of these blends by the children is greatly in excess of errors. It is also evident that omissions exceed substitutions in frequency and are more variable.

SUMMARY

Articulation data were secured by means of a test of final double reversed consonant blends administered to 273 children with cerebral palsy from six eastern states, ten northern central states, nine southern states and six western states. The following results were obtained: (1) regional differences in the articulation of these sounds were not present, (2) sex differences were not present, (3) there were low correlations between the articulations and chronological age, mental age and IQ, (4) 22% of the children were in the normal mental range, 3% were above (75% were below IQ 90 and 42% were below IQ 70), (5) no significant differences were present between spastics and athetoids, (6) paraplegics exceed quadriplegics, (7) no differences were apparent between right and left hemiplegics and (8) correct articulations of these blends by these children exceed both substitution and omission errors and omissions exceed substitutions.

Chapter 17

A Test of Triple Consonant Blends

THIS STUDY IS an attempt to restandardize Templin's Test of Triple Consonant Blends with a view to its use with cerebral palsied children. The rationale of test construction is based on the principle that a test to be used with a given population should be standardized on a sample of that population. The Templin test was designed for use with normal children. The effort here is to determine if it can be used with cerebral palsied children. The method will be to determine the reliability and validity of the test and also to make an item analysis evaluating the difficulty of the test items, their discriminating power and uniqueness.

Articulation data were collected on tape on two samples of cerebral palsied children between the ages of 5 and 16 years. There were one hundred subjects in each sample. In the first sample the data was collected in thirteen states while in the second sample they were secured in ten different states.

PROCEDURE

The Templin list of words containing triple blends was read to the subject. He was asked to repeat them one by one. The responses were taped. The two hundred subjects ranged in chronological age from 5 to 16 years with a mean of ten years. The mental age range was 3 to 12 years. The mean was 6 years, 4 months. The range of IQ scores was 26 to 116 with a mean of 77.

RESULTS

The Effect of Sex

The means and standard deviations of the scores of boys and girls for sample 1 and 11 were clustered closely around a mean of 13.0 ± 4.9.

Since the means are the same and heterogeneity of variance negligible, this may be taken as evidence of the reliability of the Templin test when used with children with cerebral palsy.

Validity of the Test

In order to determine the validity of the Templin Test when used with cerebral palsied children, the method of extreme groups was applied to the data. The usual two criteria were used: the medical diagnosis of mild and severely paralyzed children and ratings by the speech therapist of their general language ability and communicability. The articulation means of the children diagnosed by the physician as mild and severe and also the means of those rated good and poor by the therapist were compared. T-tests were applied. The mean score for the mild cases was 15.6 ± 4.0, for the severe it was 9.5 ± 4.4. The mean for the group rated good was 15.7 ± 3.6, for the poor it was 7.1 ± 3.1. All variances were homogeneous.

When the method of extreme groups was applied to the difference of the means of the articulation scores of children diagnosed as mild and severe cases, the difference of 6.1 was found

TABLE 33
Order of Difficulty of Triple Consonant Blends

Word	Blend	%
burst	-rst	51
next	-kst	56
twelfth	-lfth	56
splash	spl-	57
caged	-jd	58
spread	spr-	61
scratched	skr-	65
glimpse	-mps	66
month	-nth	67
prompt	-mpt	68
squirt	skw-	69
large	-rj	72
string	str-	77
church	-rch	77
aster	-str	81
whisker	-skr	84
number	-mbr	86
dangle	-nggl	88
twinkle	-ngkl	93

to be significant at the .001 level. The same holds true for the difference of 8.6 between the means of scores of children evaluated by the therapist as good and poor speakers. On the basis of this evidence the validity of the Templin test appears to be quite adequate.

Difficulty Range of the Items

The following table presents the triple consonant blends in order of difficulty.

The range of difficulty is from 51% to 93% with a median of 68% and a mean of 70%. Ordinarily a suitable range is from about 15% or 20% to 85% or 90%. The range of difficulty of the items of this test does not meet this criterion. This means that the items of this test are quite easy for cerebral palsied children.

Discriminating Power of the Items

Product moment correlations were used to determine the ability of items to discriminate the individual testees. If the correlations are fairly high, discriminating power is considered to be substantial. The mean r of the discriminating power of these nineteen items is .69. They range from .47 to .84. If $r = .50$ may be taken as the cutting point, then these values are quite high and the discriminating power of these triple consonant blends is satisfactory.

Uniqueness of the Items

The criterion of item uniqueness requires that the intercorrelations among the test items be low. Phi coefficients were used. The mean phi coefficient is .30 and the range extends from .13 to .53. The range rather than the standard deviation has been used because it indicates the amount of actual overlap of the uniqueness values and the discriminating powers of the items. The range for the latter is .49 to .84 with a mean of .69. The amount of overlap is minimal.

It is evident then that the test meets the criterion that the uniqueness of the items should be low while the discriminating powers should be high. The item analysis thus reveals that the items are fairly easy and that their discriminating power and their uniqueness are satisfactory.

Substitution and Omission Errors

The mean for substitutions was 1.1 ± 1.6. The mean for omissions amounted to 43.4 ± 1.6. Omissions greatly exceed substitutions of triple consonant blends.

SUMMARY

The purpose of this study was to evaluate the Templin Test of Triple Consonant Blends with a view to its usefulness with children with cerebral palsy. It was first administered to one hundred cerebral palsied children from 5 to 16 years of age in thirteen states and also to a second sample of one hundred children in ten states. The following results were obtained: sex differences are not present, the reliability of the test is evidenced by a second sample of children which confirms the finding of the first sample, the validity in terms of the method of extreme groups is adequate, the items are fairly easy for these subjects, the discriminating power of the items average .69 and range from .49 to .84. The phi correlations average .30 and range from .13 to .53, the correlations for discriminating power are higher than the uniqueness values of the items; omissions greatly exceed substitutions.

It may be concluded that this Templin test meets the criteria for the construction of a testing instrument and may be used with cerebral palsied children with the qualification that it may be found easy with some of the children.

This concludes the investigation of the problems of articulation of cerebral palsied children. The articulation of vowel sounds will be considered next.

Chapter 18

A Short Vowel Test

THIS STUDY IS concerned with the standardization of a short vowel test designed for use with children with cerebral palsy. The vowels which are included in the test are i, ɪ, ɛ, æ, ʌ, ɝ, ɑ, ɔ, o, ʊ, and u. The *e* sound has been omitted and will be consided in a forthcoming diphthong test. The sounds have been incorporated in the initial and medial positions in words. The list of words is found in Chart 4 in the Appendix.

In order to standardize the test, six criteria have been applied: (1) the reliability of the test, (2) its validity, (3) the range of difficulty of the items, (4) the discriminating power of the items, (5) their uniqueness and (6) the relation between the discriminating power and the uniqueness of the items.

PROCEDURE

The data were collected on 492 children between the ages of 3 and 16 years in twenty-three states: Arizona, Arkansas, California, Colorado, Idaho, Indiana, Iowa, Kansas, Michigan, Minnesota, Montana, Nebraska, New Mexico, North Carolina, North Dakota, Ohio, Oklahoma, Oregon, Pennsylvania, Texas, Utah, Washington and Wisconsin.

RESULTS

Reliability of the Test

The Kuder-Richardson formula No. 20 was applied to the vowels in each of the initial and medial positions. The correlation for the initial vowels yielded by the formula was .81, for the medials it was .72. In addition, test-retest reliability, an index of temporal constancy, was determined. The test was readministered to thirty-four of the subjects after an interval of twenty-one days. The coefficient of reliability was .64. This value is significant at the 1% level.

Validity of the Test

The validity of the test was determined by the method of extreme groups. Two external criteria were used, the medical diagnosis of mild and severe involvement, and the speech therapists' rating of good and poor general language ability and communicability. The means of the vowel articulation scores of the mild and severely paralyzed children were determined and found to be 18.1 and 15.0 respectively, and a t-test was applied to the difference. A similar procedure was carried out on the basis of the therapists' ratings of good and poor, where the mean for the former was 19.4, and for the latter it was 14.2. The results indicate that for the degree of involvement the probability value is at the .02 level; for the speech ratings, it is at the .001 level. These results may be taken as evidence for the validity of the vowel test.

Difficulty Range of the Items

In Table 34 the percentages of difficulty of the vowel in both the initial and medial positions are given.

It is obvious from the table that the distribution of values is unusually restricted. The range for the vowels is from 76% to 93% and the means for both positions are 88%. This is quite high and suggests that the articulation of vowel sounds by cerebral palsied children are easier than that of consonants.

TABLE 34

Difficulty Range of Vowel Sounds in Terms of Percentages

Position			
Initial		*Medial*	
U	79	ɝ	76
ɛ	86	U	86
æ	87	o	87
I	88	I	88
ɔ	88	ɑ	89
ɑ	88	ɛ	90
i	89	ɔ	90
o	90	ʌ	90
ʌ	93	æ	91
		i	91
		u	92
Mean: 88		*Mean:* 88	
Range: 79–93		*Range:* 76–92	

Discriminating Power of the Items

Another important criterion for the standardization of a test is concerned with the discriminating power of the items. It was found that the mean r is .67 and the range is from .57 to .78.

Uniqueness of the Items

It is necessary that two or more items of a test should not perform the same function. Phi coefficients were used to determine the values of item uniqueness of this test. The mean coefficient is .36 and the range is from .18 to .52.

Relation Between Uniqueness and Discriminating Power

A further consideration is that the values for the uniqueness of items must be lower than the values for their discriminating power. In this test the mean of .36 for uniqueness is much lower than that of .67 for discriminating power. Moreover, the ranges have been given for each distribution in order to show that they do not overlap. Thus the relationship between these two criteria is quite satisfactory.

SUMMARY

A test consisting of eleven vowel sounds in the initial and medial positions in words was administered to 492 children with cerebral palsy between the ages of 3 to 16 years. The data were collected in twenty-three states.

The reliability of the test was determined by a Kuder-Richardson formula. For initial vowels r = .81, for the medials r = .72. Test-retest reliability on thirty-four children with an interval of twenty-one days was .64 which was significant at the .01 level. The validity of the test was calculated by the method of extreme groups. Two determinations were made. The difference between the mean articulation scores based on the medical diagnosis of mild and severe paralysis was significant at the .02 level. The difference between the mean scores based on the speech therapists' ratings of good and poor general language ability yielded a p value of .001. The range of difficulty of the items was from 76% to 93% with a mean of 88%. The mean correlation coefficient for the discriminating power of the items was .67 and the range was from .57 to .78. The mean phi coefficient for the uniqueness of items was .36 and the range was .18 to .52. This mean is lower than that for the discriminating power and the range also is lower.

DISCUSSION

Of the six criteria used in the standardization of the vowel test—namely, its reliability, its validity, the range of difficulty of the items, their discriminating power and uniqueness, and the relation between the latter two—all are met in a satisfactory manner except the range of difficulty of the items. Children with cerebral palsy seem to articulate vowel sounds more easily than consonants; the range is from 76% to 93%. This is too restricted. The mean of 88% is too high. A preferable range might be from 10% or 15% to 85% or 90% with the mean in the neighborhood of 50%. It is also possible that the vowel sounds in the second syllable of polysyllable words would provide a wider range of the difficulties of these phonemes.

Chapter 19

Correct Status of Vowels in the Speech
of Children with Cerebral Palsy

THIS IS A REPORT on the ability of children with cerebral palsy to articulate vowel sounds. The list of vowels is found in Chart 4 (see Appendix). The report is in two parts. The aims of Part I are to determine (1) the effect of sex on vowel articulation, (2) the effect of chronological age, mental age and of the IQ, (3) the relation to the medical diagnosis, (4) the relation to the extent of paralytic involvement and (5) the relation to the degree of involvement. Part II presents data collected on additional samples of cerebral palsied children in three geographical areas—namely, the Midwest, the Mountain and the Pacific States. The purpose of this section is to check some of the findings derived from the analysis of data in Part I.

RESULTS

Part I

The Effect of Sex

Data on 134 children, seventy boys and forty-four girls, were used in this analysis. The means of the two sexes are identical, amounting to 17.1 ± 4.7. Boys and girls, therefore, may be presumed to be alike in the articulation of these vowel sounds. This result is comparable to those found in the consonantal speech of cerebral palsied children.

Relation to Chronological Age, Mental Age and IQ

The correlation of vowel scores and chronological age was .08. With mental age it was .19. With IQ it was .10. The correlations are too low for predictive purposes. In a study on the relation of these factors with ten different consonants the r values also were found to be low.

81

Substitution Errors

Comparing the errors of articulation of vowel sounds, the mean for the correct is 17.1 ± 4.3. For the substitutions it is 1.5 ± 1.1. It is obvious that the correct articulation of vowel sounds in the speech of these children greatly exceeds their substitutions. Too few omissions occurred, rendering an analysis of them futile. Not only are the above means quite different but the variability between the distribution also is large.

The Effect of Position

When the initial and medial vowel sounds are compared, the mean for the initials is 7.8 ± 2.1. For medials it is 9.4 ± 2.7. N = 114.

The difference in favor of the medials is significant at the .001 level. The variances are homogeneous.

Relation to Medical Diagnosis

In this sample there were forty-four spastics and twenty-three athetoids. A t-test was run on the difference between the means of the two groups. The means are 18.3 and 15.6. The difference of 2.7 between the means of the spastics and the athetoids is significant at the .01 level, the spastics being superior in vowel articulation. The situation however is different in the case of initial and double consonant blends where the two groups are alike.

Relation to Extent of Involvement

Again quadriplegics exhibit the lowest score and paraplegics the highest score. The values are 16.9 ± 4.9 and 18.4 ± 3.9 for paraplegics. Hemiplegics are intermediate. Their mean is 17.1 ± 5.1.

In order to determine if the differences among the means are significant an analysis of variance was done. Since F was less than 1, the differences among the three means are not significant. It is interesting, however, to note that there is a progression in mean values from quadriplegics to paraplegics similar to that previously found for consonants by those types of cerebral palsy. However in the case of consonants the differences are significant, while in the case of vowel articulation they are not.

Part II

In the second part of this study articulation data on three additional samples of children with cerebral palsy were analyzed and compared with the findings of the first part. The total number of subjects available for analysis was 395. The data were from Midwest, Mountain, and Pacific States.

Correct Vowel Scores in Three Samples

The means for the three samples are 17.3 ± 4.3, 17.7 ± 4.5 and 17.8 ± 3.8. These values confirm the mean of 17.1 ± 4.5 found in an earlier sample. The reliability of the data then appears to be firmly established.

The Effect of Sex in Three Samples

Means for boys and girls for each of the three regions were determined. The means for the six groups cluster fairly closely around a value of 17.6 ± 4.1. The differences among the six groups are not significant. The results from these three samples verify the finding of the first part of the study that sex differences in vowel articulation are negligible.

The Effect of Position in Three Samples

In Part One the mean frequency of medial vowels significantly exceeded that for initials. In this part of the study the purpose is to find if this relation holds also for the three additional samples. The means of vowels in the initial position in the three regions varied from 7.7 ± 1.8 to 8.0 ± 1.9. For the medial position they varied from 9.5 ± 2.4 to 10.0 ± 1.9. Thus the three samples confirm the first sample. This is another demonstration of the reliability of the data.

SUMMARY

This study is concerned with the ability of children with cerebral palsy to articulate vowel sounds. The aims were to determine (1) the effect of sex on vowel articulation, (2) the effect of chronological age, mental age and IQ, (3) the relation to the medical diagnosis, (4) the relation to the extent of paralytic involvement, (5) the relation to the degree of involvement, and (6) the effect of geographical regions. Four samples of children with cerebral palsy from 3 to 16 years were used in the analyses. They were from the Pacific, Mountain, and Midwest states. There were two samples from the Midwest.

In the first Midwest sample it was found (1) that the sex factor is negligible, (2) that the correlation of vowel scores with chronological age, mental age and IQ were too low for predictive purposes, (3) that correct scores significantly exceed substitutions and omissions, (4) that medial consonants significantly exceed initials, (5) that spastics significantly are superior to athetoids and (6) that there are no significant differences in the mean scores of quadriplegics, hemiplegics, and paraplegics. In the second part of the study three samples confirmed the mean value for the correct scores found in Part I. It supported the finding that the sex factor is negligible and that medial vowels significantly exceed initials. It showed regional differences in the articulation of vowel sounds by children with cerebral palsy do not exist.

Chapter 20

A Short Diphthong Test

A SERIES OF articulation tests designed for use with children with cerebral palsy included several short consonant tests, consonant blend tests and a vowel test. The present report concerns the standardization of a diphthong test. The sounds which are included are *oU, aU, eI, aI,* and *ɔI.* They have been placed in three positions in words. The list is found in Chart 8 of the Appendix.

The standardization of the test involved the attempt to meet six criteria: (1) its reliability, (2) its validity, (3) the range of difficulty of the items, (4) the discriminating power of the items, (5) their uniqueness and (6) the relation between the discriminating power and the uniqueness of the items.

PROCEDURE

Articulation data were gathered on 166 cerebral palsied children between the ages of 3 and 16 years in twelve southern and northern central states.

RESULTS

Reliability of the Test

Applying the Kuder-Richardson formula No. 20 to the diphthong scores in the initial, medial and final positions in the test words, the coefficients of reliability were .53, .64 and .51.

Validity of the Test

In order to determine the validity of the test, the method of extreme groups was used. The usual sets of extreme groups were used. In one the mean difference of articulation scores between children rated by the physician as mild or severe was calculated. The other mean difference in the scores was based on the rating of the speech therapist of very good and very poor general language ability and communicability. The difference between the means of 12.9 ± 1.9 for the mild cases and 8.6 ± 4.3 for severe is 4.3; df = 103, t = 7.24 and p = .001. The mean for the group rated very good is 13.1 ± 1.2. For the very poor it is 5.5 ± 4.2. Difference = 7.6, df = 34, t = 7.90, and p = .001.

The significance level for both calculations is .001. Thus the significant difference between the means according to the medical diagnosis as well as the general speech ratings provides evidence for the validity of the test.

Difficulty Range of the Items

The difficulty of the diphthongs for cerebral palsied children ranging from the most difficult to the least difficult for each position is given in percentages in Table 35.

It will be noted that diphthongs are fairly easy for children with cerebral palsy to articulate, the percentages being quite large. In this respect, they resemble vowels. The easiest sound is the diphthong *eI*. The range of difficulty is from 67% to 92%. If an acceptable range ordinarily would be from 15% or 20% to 85% or 90%, then the range of difficulty of diphthongs does not meet the usual criterion. The order of difficulty varies from position to position. For instance, *oU* is second in the initial column, fourth in the medial, and last in the finals.

Discriminating Power of Diphthongs

The correlation of the scores on an item with the scores of the whole test yields a value which indicates the discriminating power of an item. A necessary characteristic of correlations of

TABLE 35
Difficulty of Diphthongs in Percentages for the Three Positions

Initial	%	Medial	%	Final	%
aI	80	au	67	aU	76
oU	80	aI	78	aI	77
aU	83	ɔ	80	ɔI	81
eI	83	oU	81	eI	86
ɔI	*	eI	84	oU	92

* Not included in the initial position.

discriminating power is that they should be fairly high. The mean *r* for the discriminating power of the diphthongs is .75 and the range is from .63 to .85. These are acceptable values.

Uniqueness of the Items

The mean of these intercorrelations is .38; the range is from .12 to .65. The majority of these values are low, only two of them being above .50. Thus they meet the criterion of uniqueness.

Relation Between Discriminating Power and Uniqueness

A further requirement for the standardization of a test is that a certain relation should exist between the uniqueness of its items and their discriminating power. In other words the best test is one in which the individual items correlate highly with the test score but show relatively low intercorrelations. In the present test the mean intercorrelation is .38, while that for discriminating power is .75. The range for the uniqueness values is .12 to .65, for discriminating power it is .63 to .85, with very slight overlapping. Thus the diphthong test meets this requirement adequately. Of the six criteria for the successful standardization of a test, five of them are acceptable.

SUMMARY

A diphthong test was constructed with fourteen word items including five diphthongs in three positions in words. The diphthongs were *oU, aU, eI, aI,* and *ɔI.* The test was standardized on the basis of six criteria: (1) its reliability, (2) its validity, (3) the range of difficulty of the items, (4) the discriminating power of the items, (5) their uniqueness and (6) the relation of the discriminating power and the uniqueness of the items. Data were collected on 166 children with cerebral palsy between the ages of 3 and 16 in twelve states.

By means of a Kuder-Richardson formula it was found that the coefficients of reliability of the test were .53 for the initial position, .64 for the medials and .51 for the finals. The validity of the test was determined by the method of extreme groups. The difference between the means of articulation scores of children diagnosed by the physician as mild and severely involved was 4.3, a value significant at the .001 level. The difference between the means of scores of children rated very good and very poor in general language ability was 7.6 which was also significant at the .001 level. The range of difficulty of the diphthongs varied from 67% to 92%. This is a limited range. The discriminating power of the items varied from .63 to .95 with a mean of .75. The uniqueness of the items range from .12 to .65 with a mean of .38.

Chapter 21

Correct Status of Diphthongs

IN A PREVIOUS CHAPTER the ability of children with cerebral palsy to articulate vowel sounds was reported. The present investigation concerns the status of diphthongs in the speech of cerebral palsied children. The diphthongs are *oU, aU, eI, aI* and *ɔI*. They were placed in three positions in words. The list is given in Chart 8 of the Appendix.

RESULTS

The Effect of Sex

The means for both boys and girls was 11.2 ± 3.7. Since the standard deviations are about the same and the means are identical, no sex differences are apparent in these data. In this respect the finding is similar to that of vowels.

Relation to Chronological Age, Mental Age and IQ

The correlations of chronological age, mental age and IQ were .03, .19, and .17. The N of 64 represents the number of children common to the three categories.

The correlations between the diphthong articulation scores and chronological age, mental age and IQ accordingly are too low for predictive purposes. This result is similar to the correlation of these variables with vowel and with consonant articulation.

Relation to Right and Left Hemiplegia

When the scores of right and left hemiplegics are compared and a t-test applied, it became apparent that the difference between the means is slight. That of right hemiplegics is 11.8, while that for left hemiplegics is 10.9. It is interesting that this unexpected finding should occur again.

Relation to Extent of Involvement

The next step is to compare the means of quadriplegics, hemiplegics and paraplegics.

A progression of mean values exists from quadriplegics to paraplegics. Again quadriplegics make the lowest score. The mean is 10.3 ± 4.1. Hemiplegics come next with a mean of 11.4 ± 4.5. Paraplegics make the highest score. The mean is 12.9 ± 2.3. A similar progression has been found in the analyses of vowel and consonant sounds. In order to learn if there are significant differences among the means of the groups, an analysis of variance was done. The F value was significant at the .05 level which affords evidence that differences exist among the means of diphthong articulation of the three groups. It remains to test where the differences lie. For this purpose t-tests were run on the differences between quadriplegics and hemiplegics, between hemiplegics and paraplegics, and quadriplegics and paraplegics.

The differences between the means of the quadriplegics and hemiplegics and between the hemiplegics and paraplegics are not significant. However, the differences between the quadriplegics and paraplegics is such that the null hypothesis may be rejected.

Relation to Medical Diagnosis

In diphthong articulation the spastic cases exhibit a mean of 11.6 ± 3.5. The mean of the athetoids is 9.0 ± 5.2.

Since the variance of the two sets of scores is heterogeneous the Cochran-Cox modified t was used to determine the significance of the difference between the two means. It is indicated that the spastics are significantly superior to athetoids in the articulation of diphthongs. A similar finding occurred with vowel articulation.

The Effect of Position

The effect of the position of diphthongs in test words is indicated by a progression of values from the initial position to the final position. The mean of the initials is 3.2 ± 1.1, of the medials it is 3.9 ± 1.1 and of the finals it is 4.1 ± 1.2.

The best score made by the children in articulating these diphthongs is in the final position. This is a reversal of the situation with consonants.

Furthermore the differences in the means of diphthongs between the initials and finals are both significant at the .001 level. This then constitutes evidence that the reversal in the effect of position of diphthongs is a true one. In this it resembles the vowels where medials are significantly more prominent than initials in the speech of these children.

SUMMARY

This study is an investigation of the articulation of diphthongs by children with cerebral palsy. The diphthongs are *oU, aU, eI, aI and ɔI*. The data were collected from the speech of 166 children in twelve states. They ranged in age from 3 to 16 years.

It was found that the means for boys and girls were the same and that there is no difference in variability between the sexes. The correlations between the articulation scores for chronological age, mental age and IQ were too low for predictive purposes. For chronological age, $r = .03$; for mental age $r = .19$; for IQ, $r = .17$. No difference between the means of diphthong scores of right and left hemiplegics existed. No significant differences were found between quadriplegics and hemiplegics or between hemiplegics and paraplegics, but the difference between the means of quadriplegics and paraplegics was such that the null hypothesis may be rejected. Spastic children do better significantly than athetoids, and spastic quadriplegics are superior to athetoid quadriplegics in the articulation of diphthongs. An interesting situation exists in regard to the ability of these children to articulate diphthongs in the initial, medial and final position of words. The best score is made in the final position. The significance value lies at the .001 level. A similar result was found in respect to vowels where medials are more frequent than initials. This is a reversal of the situation with consonants where finals are not articulated as frequently as initials or medials.

Chapter 22

Replication of an Investigation of Diphthong Articulation

IN THE PREVIOUS investigation of diphthong articulation by children with cerebral palsy, it was found that the mean for their correct responses was 11.2 with a standard deviation of 3.8. The present study is an attempt (1) to replicate the first study in order to determine if it may be confirmed, (2) to learn if there are regional differences in the articulation of these sounds and (3) to determine if omission errors exceed substitutions, as is the case in consonant articulation by these children. The diphthongs are *oU, aU, eI, aI, ɔI,* the test employed in these studies is found in Chart 8 in the Appendix.

PROCEDURE

In the previous investigation, the diphthong test was administered in twelve states to 166 children from 3 to 16 years of age. In addition, it was administered to cerebral palsied children in three regions: (1) to 148 subjects in California, Oregon and Washington, (2) to 84 children in the mountain states of Arizona, Colorado, Idaho, Montana and Utah, and (3) to 88 subjects in the central states of Indiana, Michigan, Ohio, Western Pennsylvania and Texas.

TABLE 36
Replications by Regions of Diphthong Articulation of Correct, Substituted and Omitted Responses

	N	Correct		Substitutions		Omissions	
		M		M		M	
Original Study	166	11.2	3.8	1.0	1.9	0.8	1.4
Pacific	148	10.8	3.8	1.0	1.7	1.3	1.6
Mountain	84	10.7	3.7	1.1	2.1	1.5	1.8
Central	88	10.1	4.1	1.1	1.7	1.4	2.0

RESULTS

The pertinent data are given in Table 36. The table includes means and standard deviation of correct, substituted, and omitted responses by the children in four samples of diphthong articulation.

From an inspection of the table it is obvious that correct articulation of diphthongs by children with cerebral palsy exceeds substitution errors in the ratio of 10 to 1. They exceed omissions in about the same ratio.

Correct Responses

In order to determine if the difference among the means of the correct responses are significant, an analysis of variance was done. The analysis of variance indicated that the differences among the means of correct responses in the four regions are not significant. This is strong evidence of the reliability of this test for use with cerebral palsied children. It is interesting to note that this is consistent with the replications in a previous study on the correct status of vowel sounds.

Substitution and Omission Errors

It remains to find out if the replications of the original study of diphthongs yields a similar outcome in respect to substituted and omitted errors and also if the differences between the means of these two types of errors are statistically significant.

The analysis of variance yielded no evidence for significant differences between the means of substitute and omission errors. The F ration for the errors is less than 1. In this regard diphthongs differ from consonant articulation in which omissions by these children exceed substitutions. Moreover the differences among the means of substitution errors in the four samples (regions) are not significant. The p value is .20. Thus the replications confirm the result of the original investigation.

SUMMARY

This study is a replication of a previously reported investigation of diphthong articulation by children with cerebral palsy. Data on the speech of 148 children in the Pacific States, 84 in the Mountain States, and 88 in the Central States as well as 166 subjects in the original investigation were analyzed in terms of correct responses. Thus the result of the original study was corroborated. There were no significant differences among the means of substitution errors of the several samples. The same result was found also for omission errors. Moreover there were no significant differences between the substitution and omission errors. In this respect this is a different result than that found with consonants where usually omissions exceed substitutions. The frequency of correct responses of diphthongs strikingly exceeds errors in the speech of cerebral palsied children. Regional differences in the articulation of diphthongs by these children are not apparent in the data.

Chapter 23

Speech Differences Among
Cerebral Palsied Subclasses

THE PURPOSE OF this descriptive study was to investigate and summarize possible differences in speech adequacy among certain cerebral palsied subclasses. Of particular interest were the relationships of speech ability to type of condition, degree of physical involvement and chronological age of the subject. Specifically, the study examined the following three questions: (1) Were athetoid and spastic subjects significantly different with respect to the degree of speech dysfunction? (2) Was there a significant association between the degree of physical handicap and speech dysfunction among these cerebral palsied subjects? (3) Was chronological age significantly related to speech ability in this population?

PROCEDURE

A nationwide sample comprised of 497 boys and girls with cerebral palsy who were between the ages of 6 and 17 was located. At the time of their selection, the subjects were receiving services provided by such diverse facilities as hospitals, public schools and local day centers. Because of the size of the sample, it was supposed that the subjects were fairly representative of the cerebral palsied population.

Medical reports were used to determine the types and degrees of the cerebral palsied conditions. Speech ability was determined by the speech therapist who was responsible for the subject's therapy. The therapist rated the child's ability on a five-point scale.

The analysis was in terms of (1) the two types of cerebral palsy

---

Note: This chapter was conducted and written with the collaboration of Don D. Hammill.

(only two types were found in numbers sufficient to warrant analysis), (2) the three levels of degree of involvement, (3) the five speech ratings and (4) the five age levels. These data were processed on the 1604 Data Control Computer at The University of Texas according to multiple linear regression techniques described by Bottenberg and Ward (1963). A .05 level of confidence was chosen as the criterion of significance.

RESULTS AND DISCUSSION

The computed mean speech ratings by therapists and the number of cases associated with the pertinent cerebral palsied subclasses are found in Table 37 for the athetoid subjects and Table 38 for spastic subjects.

The F ratios related to the various questions raised are reported in Table 39.

In each of the comparisons reported in Table 39 the restriction was that there was no difference; for example, in comparison No. 6 the restriction being tested was that the difference between weights associated with vectors representing mild, moderate and severe diagnosed spastics was equal to 0. As the F associated with this restriction was significant at the .01 level of confidence, the hypothesis that there was no difference was not accepted.

The results are under the headings of the three proposed questions:

1. Did athetoid and spastic subjects differ significantly with respect to speech dysfunction? Apparently they did. The F testing that difference was highly significant. Furthermore, spastics were found to demonstrate speech superiority over athetoids at all levels of physical disability. (Nos. 2–4). A cursory comparison of the column totals for Table 37 and

TABLE 37
Frequency and Mean Speech Ratings for Athetoids
Age in Years

Degree	6 to 7		8 to 9		10 to 11		12 to 13		14 to 17		Total	
	f	X	f	X	f	X	f	X	f	X	f	X
Mild	9	2.3	6	3.0	4	2.8	7	3.4	5	2.2	31	2.7
Moderate	11	2.1	8	2.4	11	2.7	9	2.8	9	2.9	48	2.6
Severe	8	1.5	18	1.8	11	1.8	14	2.7	12	1.8	63	2.0
Total	28	2.0	32	2.2	26	2.3	30	2.9	26	2.3	142	2.3

TABLE 38

Frequency and Mean Speech Ratings for Spastics

Age in Years

Degree	6 to 7		8 to 9		10 to 11		12 to 13		14 to 17		*Total*	
	f	X	f	X	f	X	f	X	f	X	f	X
Mild	35	3.8	30	3.4	32	3.7	18	3.7	32	3.9	147	3.7
Moderate	31	3.8	38	3.8	17	3.8	14	3.8	23	3.5	123	3.7
Severe	25	3.0	21	2.8	17	2.6	12	2.9	10	3.8	85	3.0
Total	91	3.6	89	3.4	66	3.5	44	3.5	65	3.7	355	3.5

38 shows that spastics consistently received higher ratings than athetoids at all chronological age levels. Therapists rated the average spastic 3.5 (midway between borderline and adequate) and rated the average athetoid 2.3 (non-adequate). The observed difference is demonstrated further by the fact that 57% of the spastics were rated as having adequate speech (ratings four and five) while only 16% of the athetoids were so rated.

2. Was there a significant association between the degree of physical handicap and speech dysfunction among these cerebral palsied subjects? Among both athetoids (No. 5) and spastics (No. 6) the level of physical involvement made a significant difference in the observed speech rating. Examination of the totals of Tables 37 and 38, however, indicated that the difference was accounted for by the severe category while the mild and moderate levels had essentially the same mean rating.

TABLE 39

F Ratios Associated with Questions

Comparison Number	*Description of the Comparison*	*df*	*F*	*Signif.*
1	Athetoid-Spastic	(1,495)	104.8	.01
2	Mild (Athetoid)-Mild (Spastic)	(1,491)	17.9	.01
3	Moderate (Athetoid)-Moderate (Spastic)	(1,491)	40.2	.01
4	Severe (Athetoid)-Severe (Spastic)	(1,491)	25.9	.01
5	Mild-Moderate-Severe (Athetoid)	(2,491)	5.5	.01
6	Mild-Moderate-Severe (Spastic)	(2,491)	15.0	.01
	Age Level			
7	A-E (Mild Athetoids)	(4,467)	1.3	NS
8	A-E (Moderate Athetoids)	(4,467)	.9	NS
9	A-E (Severe Athetoids)	(4,467)	1.8	NS
10	A-E (Mild Spastics)	(4,467)	1.0	NS
11	A-E (Moderate Spastics)	(4,467)	.7	NS
12	A-E (Severe Spastics)	(4,467)	2.3	NS

3. Was chronological age significantly related to speech ability in this population? The F's (Nos. 7–12) support the proposition that subjects, regardless of chronological age, received similar speech adequacy ratings when compared with subjects as having the same condition and degree of involvement.

Theoretically one would suppose that chronological age and speech ability were highly positively correlated. This premise, however, was not substantiated by the data at hand. Two possible explanations for the finding immediately come to mind: (1) the sample was biased because older nonspeech-involved cerebral palsied youngsters were not attending the facilities from which the sample was drawn or (2) the nature of this brain condition was such that it was highly resistive to speech habilitation. The data did not permit the investigators to support either explanation, but it did suggest that further study in the evaluation of speech therapy with cerebral palsied subjects would be a valuable contribution to the literature.

SUMMARY

Speech adequacy ratings were collected on a nationwide sample of 497 boys and girls with cerebral palsy. These data were used to determine whether or not group membership with regards to type of condition, degree of physical involvement and chronological age was significantly related to speech ability. Interpretation of the statistical analyses indicated that type and degree of cerebral palsy were important factors related to speech adequacy, but chronological age was not associated with the ratings to any significant extent.

This then concludes the investigation of the articulation of cerebral palsied children based on single tests. The next step in the program is to determine the results when several of these tests are given together to the same sample of children.

Chapter 24

An Integrated Articulation Test

PROCEDURE

FOUR SHORT consonant tests and a vowel test for use with children with cerebral palsy from 3 to 16 years of age previously had been standardized, each on a separate group of children. Altogether a total of 1155 subjects were used in the five samples. For each of the tests the reliability and validity was determined. In addition the difficulty ranges of the items in each test were calculated, age progression in the scores was determined, and the discriminating power and the uniqueness of the items were found. The present study is an attempt to standardize the five tests as a whole on two groups of cerebral palsied children. Hereafter the term "part test" will be used to designate the five divisions of the entire set which in turn will be referred to as the test. The term "integrated" has been applied to the assembled tests because of the common content among the five part tests. It will be demonstrated later that the intercorrelations among them are quite high.

The test in its entirety was administered to 147 subjects. They were from speech centers, public schools and hospitals in Illinois, Indiana, Kentucky, West Virginia, Ohio, Michigan and Kansas. The test was administered again to 118 children in eight midwestern and western states in order to check the results obtained on the 147 subjects. These states were California, Idaho, Iowa, Montana, Nebraska, Nevada, Wisconsin and Wyoming. Hereafter, the first group will be referred to as sample 1 and the second as sample 2.

The purpose of the present study is to compare the results of the two samples to learn in some detail if the findings of the second sample will verify those of the first sample. The following are the specific questions to be answered: Does the general mean and standard deviation of the second sample of subjects verify the general mean and standard deviation of the first sample? Does the mean and standard deviation of the second sample of boys confirm the mean of the first sample? Does the mean of the second sample of girls support that of the first? Do the scores of boys and girls belong to the same population? Does the finding on the second sample of spastics strengthen that of the first? Are the results obtained with the second sample of athetoids consistent with the first? Are the means of the quadriplegics on the first and second samples alike? Does the same hold true for hemiplegics and for paraplegics? Do the means of mild, moderate and severely involved children on sample 2 corroborate those of sample 1? Do the means of the general speech ratings of very good, good, medium, poor and very poor on the second sample correspond to those of the first? Is the test itself a reliable and valid instrument? Do the means of initial, medial and final consonants of the second sample correspond to those of the first? Does the mean of the vowels in the initial position in the second sample confirm the mean of the first sample? Does the mean of the medial vowels in the second sample verify that of the first? What is the relation of chronological age, mental age and IQ to the articulation scores on the integrated test?

Comparisons of Sample 1 and Sample 2

The method of organizing the results of the study will be to present in a series of analyses the means and standard deviations of sample 1, of sample 2 and also of the combined samples. This will be done for a number of factors. With such a detailed treatment it will be possible to show, in terms of a number of variables, the extent to which the verification of the results of the first administration of the test may be successful.

RESULTS

Comparison of the General Means

First, the general means and standard deviations for the data of sample 1 and also of sample 2 are presented in Table 40. A significance test of the difference between the means is included in the table.

The mean for sample 1 is 63.7 and that of sample 2 is 64.3. The difference is negligible and the variances of the two distributions

TABLE 40

Means and Standard Deviations of Articulation Scores of Samples 1 and 2,
Integrated Test

	N	M	σ	diff	t	df	p
Sample 1	147	63.7	20.3				
Sample 2	118	64.3	22.2	0.6	.229	262	.80

are homogeneous. Since the null hypothesis may be accepted, the second sample furnishes evidence which verifies the results obtained with the test in sample 1. The mean for the combined samples (n = 265) is 64.0 with a standard deviation of 21.1.

The following series of analyses will furnish detailed comparisons between the two samples.

The Effect of Sex

A specific variable within which an analysis may be made is the sex factor. The question is, Does the mean of the boys' scores in a second administration of this test verify the result obtained in sample 1, and does the mean of the girls' scores in sample 2 confirm the girls' mean in sample 1? Table 41 will show the results. An analysis of variance was performed.

A cursory examination of the four means in the table reveals that they are quite alike. The analysis of variance yields a probability value of less than 1, indicating that the difference among these means is not significant. Thus there is statistical evidence that in both sexes the second sample verifies the first sample. The table provides another item of information. Since sex differences are absent the articulation scores of boys and girls in subsequent analyses may be treated as belonging to a common population.

TABLE 41

Means and Standard Deviations of Articulation Scores of Boys and Girls
in Samples 1 and 2

	N	M	σ
Boys			
Sample 1	84	63.9	21.5
Sample 2	69	66.1	22.7
Girls			
Sample 1	63	63.3	21.4
Sample 2	49	62.6	26.7

TABLE 42
Kuder-Richardson Coefficients of Reliability Consonants, Integrated Test

	Sample 1 N=147	Sample 2 N=118	Combined N=265
Initial	.93	.97	.95
Medial	.97	.96	.97
Final	.92	.94	.92

Reliability of the Observer

Over the years the author has repeatedly checked his reliability in recording the sounds of infants and of children with cerebral palsy. Agreements with other observers have averaged about 90%. This means that the error in this work amounts to about 10%.

Reliability of the Test

At this point something should be said in some detail about the reliabilities of the integrated articulation test. The question here is whether the reliabilities in the case of sample 2 support those of sample 1. If the coefficients of reliability for sample 2 are of the same size as those for sample 1, the assumption is that this constitutes confirmatory evidence of the reliability of the test.

In the first study it was reported that the Kuder-Richardson coefficients of reliability were quite high. Table 42 gives the coefficients for consonants in the initial, medial and final positions in words for both sample 1 and sample 2, and also for the combined results.

It is readily seen that all these coefficients are comparable and that all including those for the combined samples are well above r = 90. Table 43 gives the coefficients of reliability for vowel sounds in the initial and medial positions.

For vowels also the coefficients are all quite high. It appears then that the Kuder-Richardson coefficients of reliability for the second sample of vowels maintain values comparable to those of the first

TABLE 43
Kuder-Richardson Coefficients of Reliability Vowels, Integrated Test

	Sample 1 N=147	Sample 2 N=118	Combined N=265
Initial	.87	.92	.89
Medial	.89	.94	.91

sample. Moreover, it was reported in a previous study that the r for temporal constancy was .98.

Comparison of Spastics and Athetoids

The next comparison is concerned with the articulation scores made by spastic and athetoid children in two samples. For spastics the means of sample 1 and sample 2 are 66.0 and 69.8. The difference is 3.8, df = 145, and t = 1.09 and p = .30. For athetoids the mean score of sample 1 is 56.5 and for sample 2 is 50.2, difference = 6.1, df = 52, t = 0.97 and p = .30.

The null hypothesis then may be accepted. However, the variances are heterogeneous. It follows therefore that, as far as measured by the central tendency of the scores, the second sample corroborates the first but that the variabilities are unlike. A similar inference may be drawn regarding the two samples of articulation by athetoids. Moreover when the mean of the combined scores of the spastics is compared with that of athetoids the former is significantly greater than the latter.

Comparison of Quadriplegics, Hemiplegics and Paraplegics

When the scores on the integrated test of the quadriplegics, hemiplegics and paraplegics are compared, the relative standing previously reported is confirmed. The mean of the quadriplegics is 60.5 ± 22.8. Of the hemiplegics it is 67.0 ± 21.3 and of the paraplegics it is 72.3 ± 15.0. The difference of 5.3 between quadriplegics and paraplegics lies at the .001 level of confidence.

Relation to Degree of Involvement

The children in both samples were classified as mild, moderate and severe cases of involvement by the physician. The means of articulation of the mild cases of the two samples are about the same. The mean of the combined scores of the mild is 75.0 ± 9.4. The mean of the moderate samples is 68.9 ± 15.5 and the mean of the combined scores of the severe is 40.4 ± 24.1. The differences among these three means are so large as to preclude the necessity of applying an analysis of variance. It is interesting to note that the means decrease in size from mild to severe but that the standard deviations increase. This means that some severely involved children do fairly well on the test.

Effect of Right and Left Hemiplegia

The mean for right hemiplegics on this test is 65.2 ± 25.1, $N = 11$, for left hemiplegics it is 64.2 ± 22.7. $N = 8$. The standard deviations are similar indicating that the variances are homogeneous. The probability value lies at the .90 level. Thus no significant difference is apparent between right and left hemiplegics. This result is based on small Ns but it supports previous findings.

Relation to Language Ratings

Each child was evaluated by the therapist for speech intelligibility and general language ability. A five-point scale was used for this purpose. The scale steps were very good, good, medium, poor and very poor. The anchor term was "very good," which means that the child's speech corresponded to that of a normal child. The low end of the scale, very poor, means that vocalization was present but unintelligible.

The means of sample 1 and sample 2 for the children rated very good for general language ability are the same, and the standard deviations are close indicating that the variances are homogeneous. Since the difference between the means of the very good rating is only 0.1, and the variances are alike, the second sample very adequately corroborates the finding of the first sample for this category. The means for the two samples for the category "good," for "medium," for "poor," and for "very poor" each are practically the same. The variances for "poor" and "very poor" are homogeneous, but those for "good" and "medium" are heterogeneous. In the main then, in terms of this analysis, the results obtained from sample 2 substantiate those of sample 1.

The means of the combined scores of the very good rating is 79.2. For good, medium, poor and very poor the means are 75.4, 71.8, 50.5, and 31.2. They confirm previous findings.

Validity of the Test

At this point it may be desirable to report the validity of the test based on the combined data of the two samples. The method used throughout the courses of this research project for estimating the validity of the tests was the method of extreme groups. It is described by Anastasi (1955) and by Atkins (1947). Two ex-

TABLE 44
**Validity of the Integrated Articulation Test for Children with Cerebral Palsy
Using Method of Extreme Groups
Samples 1 and 2 Combined**

		Means of Medical Diagnosis			
Mild	Severe	diff	t	df	p
75.0	40.5	34.5	12.6	165	.001
		Means of Speech Ratings			
Very Good	Very Poor	diff	t	df	p
79.2	31.2	48.0	11.2	73	.001

ternal criteria were used in the study. One pair of extremes was based on the medical diagnosis of mild and severe paralytic involvement. The other was the therapists' rating of very good and very poor speech intelligibility and general language facility.

The means and standard deviations together with *t* values are presented in Table 44.

On both external criteria—that is, the medical diagnosis of mild and severe involvement and general language ability of very good and very poor—the table indicates that the difference between the means of extreme groups are significant at the .001 level. These results may be accepted as evidence for the validity of the test.

Initial, Medial and Final Consonants

A further analysis is based on the means of samples for initial, medial and final consonants in words. They are, in order, 17.3 ± 5.9, 17.0 ± 7.7, and 11.8 ± 6.3.

In regard to the combined samples 1 and 2 the initials and the medials are alike, but the mean for the final consonants is significantly lower than for either initials or medials.

The situation in regard to vowels is similar to previous findings. The mean of the combined sample of initial consonants is 7.9 ± 1.7. For medial it is 9.4 ± 2.6.

Relation to Chronological Age, Mental Age and IQ

All of the 265 cases were available for correlating chronological age at the time of administration of the articulation test. Only 178 children were given mental tests. In a previous chapter the relation of chronological age, mental age and IQ to articulation scores were reported. The correlations were quite low. In this section a similar study was done using the combined scores of the two samples.

The correlation of the articulation scores of these cerebral palsied children with chronological age is .11; with mental age it is .27 and with IQ it is .44. The coefficients of determination (r^2) respectively are 1%, 7% and 19%. These coefficients indicate the proportions of variance of articulation scores which are predictable from chronological age, mental age and IQ. The values afford scant basis for purposes of prediction. In this respect they are comparable to those previously reported.

The test will yield two kinds of information about the cerebral palsied child's articulation. It will provide the therapist with both qualitative and quantitative knowledge about the child's ability to articulate. Articulatory errors and deficits can be systematically identified and recorded. Moreover a numerical score on each part test and on the test as a whole can be obtained. With this information before her, the therapist can then plan a program for the child using any remedial method or methods available to her. After a suitable period the part tests or their alternates can be readministered. The scores of the earlier and later administrations may then be examined and compared and a precise quantitative statement may be made concerning progress. In addition qualitative improvement about the articulation of particular sounds can be noted and new misarticulations can be recorded, enabling the therapist to set up a new therapy program for the child.

The special advantage of this test is that it provides quantitative scores for comparative purposes. It may be used to measure clinical growth of the individual child or of groups of children. It also may be used to compare and evaluate clinical techniques and methods of therapy. It should aid in the measurement of articulation of children with cerebral palsy in a valid, reliable, objective fashion.

SUMMARY

An articulation test of eighty-seven items consisting of vowel and consonant sounds was administered to two samples of cerebral palsied children. The first sample included 147 children from speech centers in Illinois, Indiana, Kansas, Kentucky, Michigan, Ohio and West Virginia. The second sample included 118 children from California, Idaho, Iowa, Montana, Nebraska, Nevada, Wisconsin and Wyoming. The purpose of the present study was to compare in considerable detail the results of the two samples to determine if the findings of the second sample would verify those of the first. The following results were obtained: The general mean of the first sample was 63.7, of the second it was 64.3; the variances were homogeneous, the difference of 0.6 is not significant. The difference between the means of the boys of the two samples was not significant. The difference between the means of girls of the two samples was not significant. Coefficients of reliability of consonant sounds in the initial, medial and final positions in words were comparable in the two samples, they ranged from .92 to .97. Coefficients of reliability of vowel sounds in the initial and medial positions in words in the second sample confirmed those of the first sample, they ranged from .87 to .94. The means of scores by spastics in the first and second samples revealed no significant difference; there was no significant difference between the means of the two samples of athetoids. The mean of the second sample of articulation by quadriplegics supported that of the first sample; the same is true for hemiplegics, as well as for paraplegics. Mildly involved children make the same mean score in both samples. The variances are homogeneous, a similar situation holds for moderately involved cases and also for the severely involved. The means for the two samples of children rated very good by the speech therapist are alike and the variances are homogeneous; similar results were found for children rated good, medium, poor and very poor. The means of scores of the two samples of initial consonants in words was the same, the standard deviations were alike, a similar situation obtained for medial consonants, the means for finals were identical and the standard deviations were the same. The means for initial vowels for the two samples were alike and those for medial vowels were identical, variances were homogeneous.

Additional information yielded by combining the two samples of the study follows: Sex differences among cerebral palsied children between the ages of 3 and 16 years are not present. Athetoids made a lower mean score than spastics, the significance of the difference between means is at the .001 level. Paraplegics make a significantly higher score than either hemiplegics or quadriplegics. The mildly involved cases make the highest mean score, the moderate are next in size, and the severely involved make the lowest mean score. The combined scores of the two samples for the therapists' ratings of very good articulation was 79.2, for good it was 75.4, for medium it was 71.8, for poor 50.5 and for very poor 31.2; the variances are heterogeneous. Test validity in terms of the combined samples was determined by the method of extreme groups, the difference between the means of children diagnosed as mild and severe by the physician was significant. The same was true of children rated by the therapists as very good and very poor. The p values were at the .001 level. This may be considered evidence for the validity of the test. When the samples for each of the three positions of consonants were combined, the means of initial and medial consonants were the same, but that of finals was significantly lower than either initials or medials. In the combined samples the mean vowel score exceeds that of initials and the variances are homogeneous. The correlations of the articulation scores of these children with chronological age, mental age and IQ were .11, .27, and .44, values too small for predictive purposes.

It may be concluded from the above series of analyses that a second administration of the articulation test to a separate group of children with cerebral palsy constitutes a substantial verification of it.

Chapter 25

Difficulties of Consonant Sounds

THIS REPORT IS concerned with articulation difficulties encountered by children with cerebral palsy on consonant sounds in the initial, medial and final positions in words and with the difficulties of vowels in the initial and medial positions. The problem of articulatory difficulty of course has been investigated a number of times with various types of subjects. However, from the standpoint of speech therapy, particularly of cerebral palsied children, it may be helpful if additional light might be thrown on the problem. For this purpose the Integrated Articulation Test consisting of eighty-seven word items including thirty-five phonemes was administered to 265 children with cerebral palsy from 3 to 16 years of age. The method of administering the test, its reliability and validity have been reported earlier.

Aims of the study were to learn (1) which sounds are most difficult for the cerebral palsied child and (2) if the order of difficulty of phonemes for them was similar in the initial, medial and final positions in words. It is assumed that the most difficult sounds are those which are articulated correctly by the fewest number of children and the easiest are those which are passed by the largest number of cases. The difficulties for children with cerebral palsy of consonants in the three positions in the test words are presented in Table 45. The table lists the sounds in order of difficulty in terms of frequency of correct articulation and of percentages from the most to least difficult. There are twenty-two initial consonants, twenty-four medials and twenty-one finals in the lists. It can be seen at a glance that the median percentage of the initials is 82, for the medials it is 73 and for the finals it is 53.

It is evident from a casual examination of the table that the order of difficulty of the consonants in the three positions is not

TABLE 45
Difficulties of Consonantal Sounds in Three Positions in Words for
Cerebral Palsied Children (N = 265)

Initial	f	%	Medial	f	%	Final	f	%
ʍ	115	43	ʍ	62	23	z	92	35
ð	171	65	ʒ	133	50	θ	105	40
s	177	67	j	161	61	t	119	45
z	177	67	ʃ	163	62	ʃ	125	47
tʃ	195	74	ð	172	65	s	130	49
θ	199	75	z	181	68	v	132	50
ʃ	205	77	θ	183	69	f	133	50
dʒ	210	79	k	187	71	r	135	51
v	213	80	t	190	72	ʒ	135	51
j	213	80	r	191	72	ð	136	51
r	215	81	s	192	73	d	140	53
f	221	83	tʃ	192	73	b	140	53
k	222	84	f	193	73	g	150	57
p	227	86	dʒ	197	74	tʃ	150	57
b	228	86	ŋ	199	75	dʒ	154	58
w5	230	87	v	201	76	p	163	62
w	232	88	n	210	79	l	167	63
g	232	88	g	214	81	n	186	70
t	232	88	p	215	81	k	188	71
n	240	91	l	219	83	ŋ	199	75
d	241	91	w	219	83	m	221	83
m	243	92	d	225	85			
			b	234	88			
			m	253	95			

the same. For instance, the *s* sound ranks third in the initial position, eleventh in the medial and fifth in the final position. This means that it is difficult for cerebral palsied children to articulate *s* in the initial position, moderately difficult in the medial and not quite as difficult in the final as in the initial position. The *tʃ* sound is fifth in the initial position, twelfth in the medial position and fourteenth in the final. The *ð* sound is second in the initial, fifth in the medial and seventh in the final position. This suggests that this *th* sound is quite difficult in the initial position, less so in the medial and fairly easy in the final position. The *k* sound is thirteenth in the initial, eighth in the medial and nineteenth in the final. The consonant *t* ranks nineteenth in the initial position, ninth in the medial and third in the final. It is evident from these statements that a given consonantal sound does not maintain the same difficulty rank in all three positions.

The ʍ sound, as in the word "why," is the most difficult initial consonant for these children. Only 115 of the 265 cases or 45% successfully articulated this sound. Among the medials, as in the word "nowhere," it likewise is the most difficult consonant. Only 23% could articulate it. There is some dispute in the literature as to whether ʍ may be accepted for wh. In this study the ʍ sound when substituted for w was classed as an error. It may be noted that the consonant *m* ranks as the easiest sound in all three positions for the children.

The findings of this study on the difficulties of sounds are important for a program of therapy with children with cerebral palsy. It is of course good educational practice to begin teaching first with easy materials. The psychological effect of this approach is to enable the learner to gain confidence in his ability and to motivate him by means of initial success. A difficult learning task attempted too soon may frustrate the child and weaken or overwhelm his self-confidence.

Chapter 26

Difficulties of Consonant Sounds
In Terms of Manner, Place and Voicing

IN THE PRECEDING chapter the orders of difficulty of phonemes were determined in the initial, medial and final positions in words.

The fundamental definition of a consonant is that it is an articulate sound produced by an obstruction, narrowing or stopping of

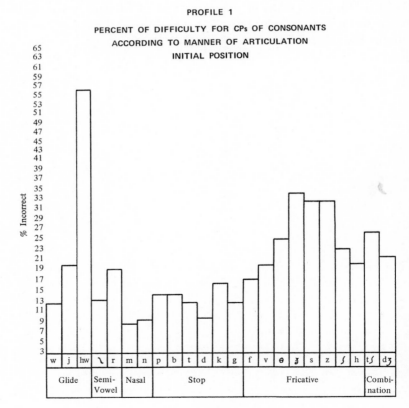

PROFILE 1

PERCENT OF DIFFICULTY FOR CPs OF CONSONANTS
ACCORDING TO MANNER OF ARTICULATION
INITIAL POSITION

PROFILE 2

PERCENT OF DIFFICULTY FOR CPs OF CONSONANTS
ACCORDING TO MANNER OF ARTICULATION
MEDIAL POSITION

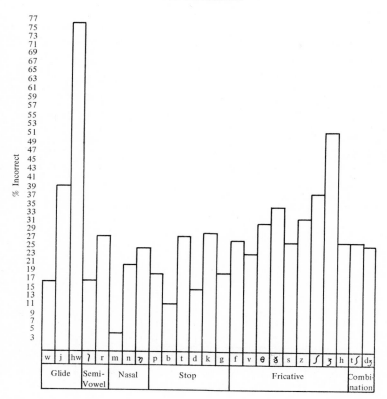

the breath stream in the oral passage. Three supplemental definitions are implicit in this statement. The consonant may be further
defined according to manner of articulation, place of articulation
and voicing. The present study is concerned with an analysis of the
consonant sounds of cerebral palsied children in terms of these
three criteria in each of the three positions of consonants in test
words. The 265 cerebral palsied children from 6 through 16 years
of age were tested using the Integrated Articulation Test.

For the purpose of the present study the norms of the previous
report have been converted from percent of correct responses to

PROFILE 3

PERCENT OF DIFFICULTY FOR CPs OF CONSONANTS
ACCORDING TO MANNER OF ARTICULATION
FINAL POSITION

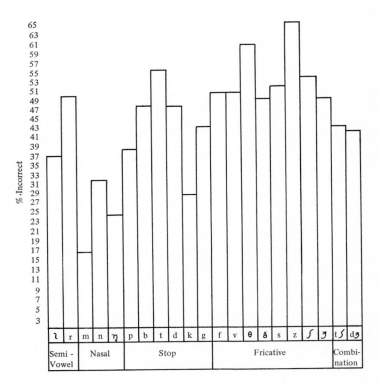

percent of incorrect responses. The converted percents have been presented in the form of profiles. The consonant sounds and their classifications are indicated on the abscissas and the percent of incorrect responses on the ordinates. Thus in profile 1 the consonant *w*, a glide, occurs with a value of 12%, the *m* sound, a nasal, has a value of 8%. These values represent the percentage of the 265 children with cerebral palsy who had difficulty with these phonemes in the initial position according to manner of articulation. Profiles 2 and 3 indicate the difficulties for manner of articulation when the sounds are in the medial and final positions.

PROFILE 4

PERCENT OF DIFFICULTY FOR CPs OF CONSONANTS
ACCORDING TO PLACE OF ARTICULATION
INITIAL POSITION

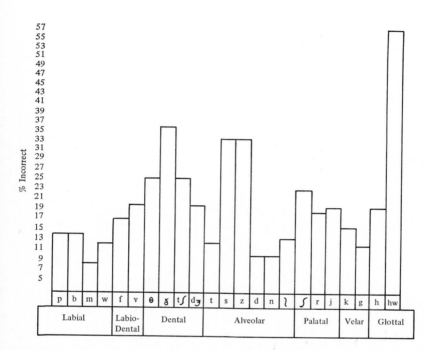

The next six tables give the profiles for place of articulation and for voicing. In profiles, 7, 8 and 9 the pairs of voiced and voiceless items are represented by blank and cross-hatched columns. The blank columns represent the percents of voiceless consonants, the cross-hatching represents the voiced sounds. It is apparent from a casual inspection of these profiles that the percents of difficulty in the final positions consistently exceed those for the initial and medial positions. The difference was found to be statistically significant. A score sheet is provided by which the articulation status of a child may be summarized.

Order of Difficulty

The values in the tables are calculated in the following manner.

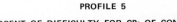

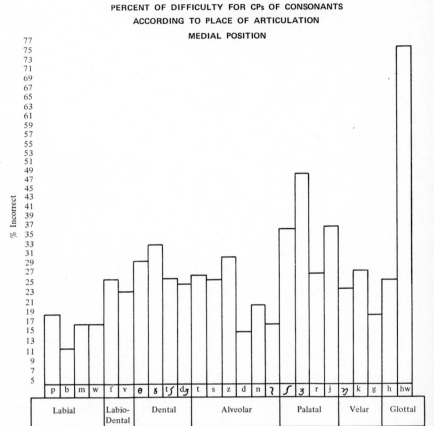

For instance in Table 46 the total percentage of the three glides in the initial position amounts to 89. The mean percent rounded then is 30. The means for the remaining categories have been calculated similarly.

Table 46 gives the orders of difficulty in each of the three positions in words for the several categories of consonants according to manner of articulation.

The table may be read as follows: of 265 cerebral palsied children, 9% have difficulty with nasal consonants in the initial position, 20% in the medial and 25% in the final position. It will be

PROFILE 6

PERCENT OF DIFFICULTY FOR CPs OF CONSONANTS
ACCORDING TO PLACE OF ARTICULATION
FINAL POSITION

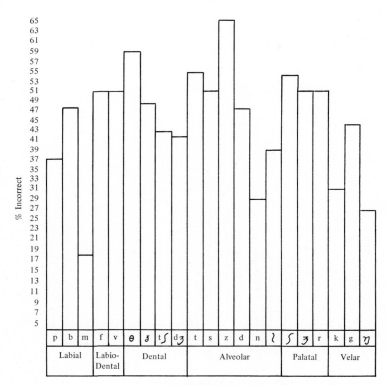

TABLE 46
Order of Difficulty According to Manner of Articulation

Initial	Mean %	Medial	Mean %	Final	Mean %
Nasal	9	Stop	20	Nasal	25
Stop	13	Semivowel	23	Semivowel	42
Semivowel	16	Nasal	26	Combination	43
Combination	24	Combination	27	Stop	44
Fricative	29	Fricative	33	Fricative	53
Glide	30	Glide	44	Glide	—

noted that the nasal category presents the least difficulty to cerebral palsied children in the initial and final positions while the fricatives and glides are the most difficult for them in all three posi-

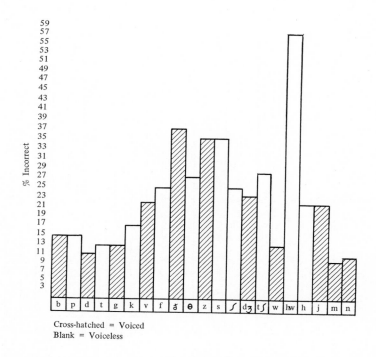

Cross-hatched = Voiced
Blank = Voiceless

tions. Stops appear to be least difficult in the medial position. Semivowels and combinations vary somewhat among the three positions.

Table 47 shows the orders of difficulty for consonants in three positions according to the place of articulation.

It is apparent that in terms of place of articulation the labials are easiest for these children and the dentals and glottals are the most difficult. Velars shift in degree of difficulty from the initial position to the final position becoming increasingly difficult. In the medial and final positions there are quite large increases in difficulty over the initial position.

TABLE 47
Order of Difficulty According to Place of Articulation

Initial	Mean %	Medial	Mean %	Final	Mean %
Labial	12	Labial	16	Labial	33
Velar	14	Alveolar	23	Alveolar	48
Palatal	18	Velar	24	Labiodental	51
Labiodental	19	Labiodental	26	Palatal	52
Alveolar	19	Dental	29	Velar	92
Dental	27	Palatal	39	Dental	99
Glottal	39	Glottal	52	Glottal	—

Table 48 presents the order of difficulty of consonants according to voicing and position in words.

There is a tendency in this sample of cerebral palsied children for the voiceless consonants to exceed the voiced in percent of difficulty.

Use of the Profiles and Score Sheet

When a new cerebral palsied case appears in the clinic, the first task is to evaluate the child's articulation with the Integrated Articulation Test. Then the errors according to place, manner and voicing for each sound should be determined. From these data a score sheet for each child may be used to record his errors. In Chart 9 of the Appendix is found the form of the score sheet. It is constructed so that each consonant and its category according to place, manner and voicing may be checked. The score sheet will provide information of the difficulty status of the child and will reveal where his severest problems lie.

Inspection of the profiles reveals, with a few exceptions, a tendency towards a fairly close concentration of the percents of difficulty among the consonants within each category. The most

TABLE 48
Order of Difficulty of Voiced and Voiceless Consonants

	Initial	Medial	Final
	Mean %	Mean %	Mean %
Voiced	18	25	43
Voiceless	25	32	47

PROFILE 8

**PERCENT OF DIFFICULTY FOR CPs OF
VOICED AND VOICELESS CONSONANTS
MEDIAL**

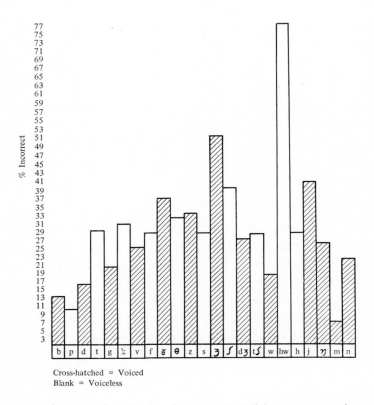

Cross-hatched = Voiced
Blank = Voiceless

pronounced exception is the *hw* sound. This concentration suggests a somewhat different approach to the practice of therapy.
It is frequently the practice in therapy to concentrate on the
improvement of one sound at a time. The profiles suggest instead
the advisability of giving simultaneous therapy on a group of
phonetically similar sounds. If for instance the score sheet reveals
that the difficulty is mainly in the production of palatal sounds,
it may be profitable for the therapist to work on several of these
sounds simultaneously instead of only one of them. Learning to
place the tongue on the palate in this instance might better be

PROFILE 9

PERCENT OF DIFFICULTY FOR CPs OF
VOICED AND UNVOICED CONSONANTS
FINAL

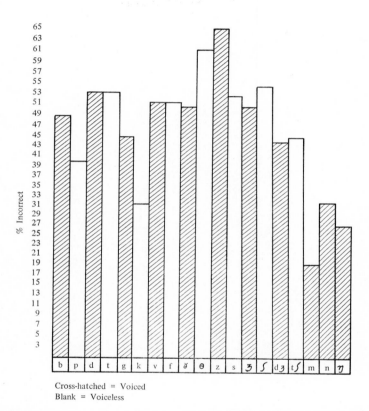

Cross-hatched = Voiced
Blank = Voiceless

accomplished by practicing several palatal sounds because the tongue movement among them is quite similar. Carry-over of the improved production of the sounds to spontaneous speech in this manner may likewise be facilitated.

The above remarks refer to one of the phonetic categories according to place of articulation. If the problem is rather with articulation according to manner and the difficulty is perhaps with the fricatives, the above remarks would be pertinent to this as well as to other categories.

CHART 9

Score Sheet According to Place, Manner and Voicing

Place		I	M	F		Manner		I	M	F		Voicing	Voiced I	M	F
Labial	p	—	—	—	Glide	w	—	—	—		θ	—	—	—
	b	—	—	—		j	—	—	—		d	—	—	—
	m	—	—	—		hw	—	—	—		g	—	—	—
	w	—	—	—	Semi-Vowel	l	—	—	—		v	—	—	—
Labio-Dental	f	—	—	—		r	—	—	—		ð	—	—	—
	v	—	—	—	Nasal	m	—	—	—		z	—	—	—
Dental	θ	—	—	—		n	—	—	—		ʒ	—	—	—
	ð	—	—	—		ŋ	—	—	—		dʒ	—	—	—
	tʃ	—	—	—	Stop	p	—	—	—		w	—	—	—
	dʒ	—	—	—		b	—	—	—		j	—	—	—
Alveolar	t	—	—	—		t	—	—	—		ŋ	—	—	—
	s	—	—	—		d	—	—	—		m	—	—	—
	z	—	—	—		k	—	—	—		n	—	—	—
	d	—	—	—		g	—	—	—			Voiceless I	M	F
	n	—	—	—	Fricative	f	—	—	—		p	—	—	—
	l	—	—	—		v	—	—	—		t	—	—	—
Palatal	ʃ	—	—	—		θ	—	—	—		k	—	—	—
	ʒ	—	—	—		ð	—	—	—		f	—	—	—
	r	—	—	—		s	—	—	—		θ	—	—	—
	j	—	—	—		z	—	—	—		s	—	—	—
Velar	k	—	—	—		ʃ	—	—	—		ʃ	—	—	—
	g	—	—	—		ʒ	—	—	—		tʃ	—	—	—
	ŋ	—	—	—		h	—	—	—		hw	—	—	—
Glottal	h	—	—	—	Combination	tʃ	—	—	—		h	—	—	—
	hw	—	—	—		dʒ	—	—	—					

Finally the use of the checklist according to manner and place and voicing together with the record of errors such as substitutions, omissions, distortions and additions secured by means of the Integrated Articulation Test should give a complete picture of the status of the articulation of the cerebral palsied child.

Chapter 27

The Applicability of an Articulation Test with Mentally Retarded Children

THE PRESENT STUDY is a statistical evaluation of the Integrated Articulation Test when administered to a different population, specifically to mentally retarded children who do not have cerebral palsy.

It is a fundamental principle of test construction that a test should be standardized on a sample of the population of subjects with which the test is to be used. It is known that many cerebral palsied children also are mentally retarded. This suggested the possibility that the test might also be used with mentally retarded children. It may be of interest to know then, if this test, designed for use with cerebral palsied subjects, would meet the several criteria of test construction when it is administered to mentally retarded children. The purpose of the present study then is to determine the possibility of the use of the test with mentally retarded children and to learn what are its advantages and limitations as a measuring instrument of the articulatory status of this group of children.

For the purpose of this study the term "mental retardation" is defined as mental functioning below IQ 80. It is customary to consider an IQ of 70 as the upper limit of mental retardation. The justification for using IQ 80 as the upper limit rather than 70 is as follows. The articulation scores of three IQ levels—51 to 60, 61 to 70, 71 to 80—are about the same. It is not until the IQ level of 81 to 90 that the scores increase significantly.

PROCEDURE

One hundred and sixty-two mentally retarded children were given the Integrated Articulation Test. They were from 3 to 16 years of age from five states—California, Idaho, Michigan,

Nebraska and Wyoming. The mean chronological age of the children was 10.6 years. The range was 3 years to 15 years, 8 months. The mean mental age was 6.6 years with a range of 2 years, 7 months, to 12 years, 8 months. No effort was made to distinguish among the various types of mental retardation.

RESULTS

Reliability of the Test

Table 49 gives the Kuder-Richardson coefficients of reliability for the test sounds in the initial, medial and final positions for consonants and vowels as determined on the sample of mentally retarded children.

It is seen that four of the five coefficients are fairly high; the value for final consonants is low.

Validity of the Test

The method of extreme groups was used to estimate the validity of the test. The two extreme groups are the educable mentally retarded children with IQ between 51 and 80, and the trainables with IQ between 25 and 50. For the purpose of determining the difference between the groups and its significance there were available 108 educables and 34 trainables. The essential data are included in Table 50.

When the difference between the means of the two extreme groups is subjected to a test the table shows it to be highly significant in favor of the educables. Moreover the variance of the trainables is much greater than that of the educables. Thus the two groups differ in regard to their central tendencies and also in regard to their variabilities. In terms of the method of extreme groups, this result may be taken as evidence for the validity of the test when used with mentally retarded children.

TABLE 49
Kuder-Richardson Coefficients of Reliability of the Integrated Test
When Used with Mentally Retarded Children

Positions	Consonants	Vowels
Initial	.91	.75
Medial	.86	.91
Final	.55	*

*There are no final vowels in the test.

TABLE 50
Validity of the Integrated Test When Used with Mentally Retarded Children

Groups	M	σ	diff	t	df	p
Educables	76.3	7.8				
Trainables	69.2	19.2	7.1	3.35	140	.001

Uniqueness of the Items

The items of a test should be functionally unique. This means that two or more of its items should not perform the same function. If the intercorrelations among the items generally are low, it may be assumed that the criterion of uniqueness has been met. Phi coefficients were used to determine the values.

If a cutting off correlation of .50 is taken as a point below which uniqueness values should fall, the criterion of uniqueness is fairly adequately met by the items of the test. The general mean for consonants is $r = .25$, for vowels it is $r = .33$. However, there are some exceptions. There are twenty-one correlations in a total of 250 which exceed the cutting value of $r = .50$ whereas 229 of them are below this value. Thus the mean of the correlations for uniqueness is low and the range of each in the main also is low.

Discriminating Power of the Items

The discriminating power of an item is measured by correlating the scores of the item with the scores of the whole test. The general mean for consonants is $r = .55$. This value is higher than that of .25 for uniqueness. For vowels the two values are .50 and .27.

Difficulty Range of the Items

The difficulty of a sound is defined in terms of the percent of subjects who articulate it correctly. The sound with the smallest percent of correct responses is considered the most difficult and the one with the highest is the easiest. The range of difficulty for mentally retarded children on the Integrated Articulation Test is 23% to 99%, for vowels it is 93% to 99%.

An acceptable range of difficulty for the items of a test is 15% or 20% to 85% or 90%. It is obvious that this range is fairly well approximated by the consonants, but the range of vowel sounds is too narrow.

Order of Difficulty

The data of Table 51 yields information about the order of difficulty of articulation by mentally retarded children. It is interesting to note that the order of difficulty of consonants varies with the position in the test words. The *r* sound ranks sixth in the initial position, ninth in the medial and sixteenth in the final position. The consonant *v* is fifth in the initial, fourteenth in the medial and sixth in the final position. Other illustrations are evident in the table. The *s* sound is ninth in the initial position, eleventh in the medial and seventh in the final. The *z* sound is third in the initial, tenth in the medial and fourth in the final position. Thus it is evident that there is no consistency among consonantal sounds from one position to another. Vowel sounds are so close together in value that the order of difficulty for the mentally retarded is meaningless.

TABLE 51
Consonant Difficulty with Mentally Retarded Subjects
Integrated Test

Initial	f	%	Medial	f	%	Final	f	%
ʌ	82	51	ʌ	37	23	z	666	41
ð	110	68	ʒ	101	62	ʒ	75	46
s	139	86	ð	132	81	g	83	51
θ	144	89	ʃ	135	83	t	86	53
v	146	90	j	137	85	θ	87	54
r	149	92	⊖	137	85	v	93	57
tʃ	151	93	k	140	86	s	95	59
ʃ	152	94	z	143	88	p	97	60
s	153	94	r	145	89	d	100	62
dʒ	154	95	t	146	90	b	104	64
w	157	97	s	148	91	ð	108	67
p	157	97	f	148	91	d	110	68
ʃ	157	97	n	149	92	f	116	73
ɺ	158	98	v	150	93	ʃ	118	73
t	158	98	ŋ	153	94	tʃ	120	74
f	159	98	tʃ	153	94	r	123	76
g	160	99	ɺ	154	95	ɺ	133	82
d	160	99	dʒ	154	95	k	134	83
n	160	99	d	154	95	n	151	93
k	161	99	w	156	96	m	151	93
m	161	99	g	158	98	ŋ	153	94
b	161	99	b	159	98			
			m	159	98			
			p	161	99			

Of further interest is the finding that the order of difficulty of consonants by mentally retarded children is unlike that for cerebral palsied children. (See Table 45.)

Relation to Chronological Age, Mental Age and IQ

The coefficients of correlation of the articulation scores with chronological age, mental age and IQ are in the order of .26, .29 and .33.

These coefficients may be evaluated by means of the index of determination which is the square of r. It indicates the proportion of the variance of one variable which is accounted for by the other variable. The r^2s are .07, .08 and .11. The r^2s reveal that the influence of these three variables on articulation is not very strong. This is consistent with the result obtained with cerebral palsied children.

SUMMARY

An integrated articulation test originally constructed for use with children with cerebral palsy was administered to 162 mentally retarded children without cerebral palsy. The purpose was to see how a test designed for use with cerebral palsied children might be used with mentally retarded children. The data were collected on recording tape in the states of California, Idaho, Michigan, Nebraska and Wyoming. The mean chronological age was 10.6 years, the range being 3 to 16 years. The mean mental age was 6.6 years with a range of 2 years to 12 years, 8 months.

The reliability of the consonants in three positions was .91 for initial consonants, .86 for medials and .55 for finals. The reliability of the vowels was .75 for initials and .91 for medial vowels.

The validity was determined by the method of extreme groups utilizing the educables and trainables as the extremes. The difference between the means of the groups was significant at the .001 level. The phi coefficients of correlation of the items of each of the part tests were low whereas the coefficients of correlation for the discriminating power of the items of the part tests were higher than those for uniqueness. There was considerable overlap of the ranges of the uniqueness and discriminating values. The range of difficulty of the items was from 23% to 99% for consonants. For vowels it was 93% to 99% indicating that vowel sounds were quite easy for mentally retarded children to master. The orders of difficulty of consonants and for vowels in the initial, medial and final positions in words were found to vary. Correlations of the articulations of the subjects with chronological age, mental age and IQ were low. It may be concluded that the Integrated Articulation Test is not as precise a measuring instrument with mentally retarded children as with cerebral palsied subjects. Although this test may be used for an evaluation of the articulation of mentally retarded children, the results obtained from these subjects should be interpreted with caution.

Chapter 28

A Short Articulation Test for Use with Mentally Retarded Children

THIS STUDY IS concerned with the standardization of a short consonant test.* The specific problem investigated is What is the status of the articulation of difficult consonantal speech sounds by a group of educable mentally retarded and a group of trainable mentally retarded? The terms "educable" and "trainable" retarded are at present used extensively in the public schools. They are generally accepted in the area of special education. The two terms are used here for the sake of consistent terminology. An educable group is usually operationally defined as having IQ scores that fall between 50 and 80. The trainable group is usually defined as having IQ scores that fall between 25 and 50.

The articulation disorders of the group of forty-one educable retarded children are compared with a group of twenty-three trainable retarded children and also with a matched group of forty-one children with normal intelligence. The test is based on ten difficult consonants. Each consonant is presented in the initial position of a word, in the medial position, and in the final position. The ten consonants were common to lists of the most difficult sounds reported in the literature for various populations.

The study investigated the following questions: (1) Sex differences: Are there differences between the sexes in the articulation of difficult consonants? (2) Group differences: Do the trainable, educable and normal groups show differences in ability to articulate the consonants? (3) Positions of consonants: Are errors equally numerous in the initial, medial and final positions of words? (4) Types of errors: Are substitution or omission errors more frequent? Do the retarded groups differ? (5) Order of dif-

---

* Constructed by Dale O. Irwin

ficulty: What is the order of difficulty of the ten consonants for the two retarded groups? (6) Relationships of articulation with chronological age, mental age and IQ: Are these variables related to articulation and which variable shows the highest relationship with articulation?

PROCEDURES

Selection of the Consonants

In order to determine which consonants should be selected for use in this study, an analysis of reports in the literature was made. A number of studies have ranked consonants in the order of difficulty for various samples of subjects. Powers (1957) reported that nine consonants gave difficulty for normal schoolchildren, and seven gave difficulty to college freshmen. Fairbanks (1940) indicated the twelve most difficult sounds for adults and children. Roe and Milisen (1942) listed ten defective consonants in the speech of schoolchildren in the first through sixth grades. Bangs (1942) listed six consonants frequently omitted in the speech of retarded children. Van Riper (1947) included ten of the most frequently misarticulated consonants in the speech of young children. Saylor (1940) found nineteen sounds defective in the speech of students in grades eight to ten. Karlin and Strazzulla (1952) determined the nine most defective sounds in the speech of three-to fourteen-year-old mentally deficient children. Spriesterbach, Darley and Rouse (1956) found that nine consonants were difficult to articulate by cleft palate children.

The selection of ten consonants from these lists were based on a tally of the sounds common to them. The number of consonants was limited to ten because that was approximately the number usually reported in literature. According to the tally, the ranking from most to least difficult is as follows: *s, z, dӡ, tʃ, ⊖, ʃ ð, r, t* and ļ. A comment should be made concerning the inclusion of the ļ sound. The sounds ӡ and ʍ rank ahead of it in the tally, but the former is not found in the initial position in words and the latter does not occur in the final position, but ļ is found in all three positions. Moreover, both Fairbanks and Bangs include it in their lists.

Having selected the ten sounds for testing purposes, the next problem was to select appropriate words to illustrate them in the three positions. The principle of selection of the words was the agreement by three therapists experienced with the articulation of speech defective children that the words in general were within the vocabulary limitations of this type of child. After the words were selected in this manner, they were placed in a randomized order. The list of words with the ten consonants placed in the initial, medial and final positions appears in Chart 10 in the Appendix.

Administration and Scoring of the Test

The test was administered to the subjects individually. Dale Irwin administered the test to the educable retarded group and to the normal group. A competent tester administered the test to the trainable retarded group. Each subject was asked to repeat each word after listening to the tester say it. The responses to the 30-item test were recorded on tape. This recording made it possible to listen to each word several times in case there was doubt as to the classification of the consonant being articulated.

The responses, as read from the tape, were classified by a check mark on an individual record form. The categories were correct, substituted, omitted, distorted, added, no response and neutral. The primary interest was in the first three categories. The categories of added, neutral, no response and distorted were included to help classify any unusual responses obtained.

Determination of Observer Reliability

Reliability was established by transcribing one hundred records of twenty-three cerebral palsied children and by transcribing fifty-seven records of ten mentally retarded children. The two observers agreed upon the classification of the consonants in 95% of the records.

RESULTS

The Effect of Sex

The mean score of educable boys was 24.4, for the girls it was 26.8. The girls scored higher than the boys. The test between the means of the sexes gave evidence that the null hypothesis may be accepted: t = 1.13, df = 39, p = .20.

The mean score of trainable boys was 19.9, for the girls it was 22.8. This group also showed a tendency for the girls to score higher than the boys. Again the value of the *t* did not warrant rejecting the null hypothesis; t = 1.42, df = 21, p = .20.

Since the sexes in both groups did not differ significantly, the two sexes within each group are combined for further analysis.

Differences Among Trainable, Educable and Normal groups

The differences between the groups were all statistically significant when compared on the t-test. The *t* value for the educable-trainable groups was 2.55, df = 62. This value is significant at the .02 level.

Inspection of Table 52 also reveals that the two retarded groups were equally variable. The standard deviation of the normal group reflects the extremely skewed distribution of scores. In fact, this group made so few errors that analysis of the errors would not be worthwhile. Because of the wide difference in the variability between the normal and educable groups the Cochran-Cox Modified t-test was used. The obtained *t* was 4.47. The modified t.01 was 3.19. Since 4.47 > 3.19 the difference between the means was significant.

The Effect of Position of Consonants in the Words

The mean of correct scores in the initial, medial and final positions for the educable retarded children was 9.66, 8.80 and 7.66. An analysis of variance and t-tests revealed that the differences between the initial-final positions and the medial-final positions were significant, but the difference between the initial-medial positions was not. A similar result occurred with the trainable group. The occurrence of more articulation errors in the final position of a word holds for both the educable mentally

TABLE 52
Differences Among Groups on Correct Score

Groups	N	Mean	SD
Normal	41	29.67	.80
Educable	41	25.12	6.36
Trainable	23	21.17	4.83

retarded group and the trainable mentally retarded group.

The means for the trainable and educable groups in the initial and medial positions are about the same. In contrast, the trainable group scored lower than the educable in the final position. The difference between the means is 2.86. The *t* value for this difference is 4.03, df = 62, which is significant at the .001 level. It appears then that in terms of mean total score, the differences between the two groups are largely accounted for by differences in the final position.

Types of Errors

The educable retarded group had more substitution errors than omission errors. The corresponding means are 3.6 and 3.1. The *t* value for related measures between the means is 4.48, df = 40. The difference is significant at the .001 level. The trainable retarded group made more omission errors than substitution errors. The means are 1.2 and 5.4. The *t* value between these two means is 4.14, df = 22. This also is significant at the .001 level.

The mean number of substitution errors between the two groups is about the same. However, the trainable group had significantly more omission errors than did the educable group. The *t* value between the two groups on omission errors is 6.62, df = 63. This is significant at the .001 level. The standard deviations are of a size which questions the reliability of the means.

Order of Difficulty of the Consonants

The difficulty of each consonant was determined by dividing the number of errors for the consonant by the total number of errors for all consonants. The percentages are used to rank the consonants from one, the most difficult, to ten. The forty-one educable retarded children made a total of 190 errors. The trainable group made a total of 192 errors.

It will be noted that the rankings of the two groups are dissimilar.

Relationship among Articulation, Chronological Age, Mental Age and IQ

The coefficient of correlation of articulation and mental age was .30. With chronological age it was −.01. With IQ it was .53.

TABLE 53
Difficulty of Consonants According to Educable and Trainable Subjects

Educable		Sounds	Trainable	
Rank	%		Rank	%
6	10.3	s	7	7.8
5	11.0	z	4	11.5
8	8.3	dʒ	2	12.5
4	11.4	tʃ	6	9.9
1	16.1	θ	5	10.5
2	13.0	ʃ	8	7.8
3	12.0	ð	1	14.6
9	5.5	r	10	6.7
10	4.1	t	3	11.5
7	8.1	l	9	5.8

The Pearson product moment correlation between articulation score and mental age is significant at the .05 level. The correlation between the articulation score and IQ is significant at the .01 level. On the basis of the size of the correlations it appears that IQ is the better predictor of articulation scores.

DISCUSSION

Ability to articulate consonants appears to be related to intellectual factors. Comparison of the normal, educable and trainable retarded shows statistically significant differences among the means of the articulation test. The educable retarded and the normal group were matched on socioeconomic ratings. Consequently, the differences between these groups cannot be attributed to home background. Since both groups attended public schools, the differences are not attributable to different formalized education. The significant differences between the educable and the trainable groups are more open to speculation. Many of the trainable were institutionalized, so the general speech environment may have been more austere.

The two retarded groups can be differentiated on the type of errors they made. The educable group made more substitution errors than omission errors. The trainable group made more omission errors than substitution errors. Moreover, they were primarily made in the final position. This reversal of the type of error between the two groups indicated that the articulation status of the two groups is not identical. The articulation status of the educable group is more like the normal group. The differences are those of quantity. The articulation status of the trainable group differs both quantitatively and qualitatively. These results demonstrate the necessity for limiting and defining the types of mentally retarded children used in research. If the results of this investigation can be generalized to all retarded children, then the efforts of speech therapists must take into account the degree of retardation. Articulation problems would vary according to the degree of retardation.

SUMMARY

This study investigated the ability of mentally retarded children to articulate difficult consonants. Ten consonants were selected from the literature which were considered to be the most difficult to articulate. The consonants were utilized in words which placed them in the initial, medial and final positions. These words were administered to a group of trainable mentally retarded children, a group of educable mentally retarded children and a group of normal children. The latter two groups were matched on the basis of age levels and socioeconomic ratings. The following results were obtained: (1) The girls in both the retarded groups exceeded the boys on mean correct scores, but the differences were not significant. (2) The three groups were differentiated on their ability to articulate difficult consonants. The higher the IQ level of the group, the higher the mean correct score. These differences were all statistically significant. (3) The normal group made too few errors to make analysis of positional and type of errors possible. The educable group was characterized by errors in all positions, with a statistically significant trend for the errors to be in the final position. (4) The educable group made significantly more substitution errors than omission errors. The trainable group made significantly more omission errors than substitution errors. (5) The following was the order of difficulty for the consonants for the two groups: for trainables—ə, dʒ, t, z, ⊖, tʃ, s, ʃ, ḷ, r; for educables—⊖, ʃ, ə, t, z, s, ʃ, dʒ, r, t. (6) The scores of the articulation test of educable group correlated with mental age .30, with chronological age −.01 and with IQ .53.

Chapter 29

Replication of the Short Articulation Test
with Cerebral Palsied Children

I N THE PRECEEDING STUDY on the ability of retarded children to articulate difficult consonantal sounds, a word list including ten difficult consonants was constructed and standardized on a group of trainable mentally retarded children and a group of educable mentally retarded.

PROCEDURE

The present study is an attempt to restandardize the short articulation test on a group of children with cerebral palsy and is one of a series of short articulation tests for use with this type of child. It is intended as a quick consonant screening test. The test was administered verbally to 333 children with cerebral palsy who ranged in age from 3 to 16 years.

RESULTS

Reliability of the Test

In order to determine the reliability of this test four methods were used. They are (1) observer reliability, (2) Kuder-Richardson's method of rational equivalence, (3) test-retest reliability and (4) parallel form reliability.

Determinations of observer reliability were made on one hundred records of twenty-two children with cerebral palsy and fifty-seven records of ten mentally retarded children. The mean agreements are 95% and 96%. Thus observer reliability is quite adequate.

The Kuder-Richardson formula No. 20 was used to determine the internal consistency of the test. It was applied separately to the consonant data in the initial, medial and final positions in the test words. The correlation values were respectively .86, .87 and

.86. This formula, however, does not measure diurnal variation. Therefore the test-retest method of determining reliability also was used. This method yields a coefficient of temporal stability. After an interval of twenty-one days, thirty-four children were retested. The coefficient of correlation was .87. The correlation of .87 means that after an interval of three weeks this test gives fairly reliable results with children who have cerebral palsy.

A parallel forms reliability also was determined. The procedure in administering the forms was as follows. First one form was given to each of 111 subjects followed immediately by a list of materials differing in content. The second form (see Chart 11 in Appendix) was then administered. The purpose of interposing foreign material was to take advantage of the factor of retroactive inhibition. If two parallel forms are administered successively, memory of the first form presumably may influence performance on the second. The presence of foreign material between the two forms, by the principle of retroactive inhibition, should reduce the memory effect. Moreover the fact that the second form of the test was built with a different set of words should also tend to obviate any carry-over from the first form. In administering the tests the forms were alternated from subject to subject. The r for the parallel forms was .85. It should be pointed out that three conditions should be met in equivalent form reliability. The means of the two administrations should be alike, the variances should be homogeneous, and the correlation should be fairly high. This constitutes the definition of equivalent test forms. The three conditions have been met in this study.

In general, on the basis of the four above analyses, the reliability of the test appears to be satisfactory. It is interesting that the three kinds of reliability yield about the same coefficient.

Validity of the Test

The validity of the test was determined by the method of extreme groups. Two different external criteria were used in selecting the extreme groups. The first was the medical diagnosis of mildly and severely involved children. The difference between the means of the articulation scores of these groups was evaluated by a t-test. The second external criterion was the speech therapist's

TABLE 54

**Validity of a Test of Ten Consonants for Children with Cerebral Palsy
Using Method of Extreme Groups**

Mean for Mild		Mean for Severe	σ	diff	t	df	p
Medical Diagnosis							
22.5	6.1	15.9	9.4	6.6	5.59	193	.001
Therapists' Ratings							
Mean for Good		Mean for Poor	σ	diff	t	df	p
24.7	7.2	11.5	8.0	13.2	13.1	248	.001

rating of the child's general language ability and communicability. The difference between the mean articulation scores of the children rated as good and poor also was subjected to a t-test. Available for the former analysis were 84 mildly involved children and 111 severely involved children, and for the second analysis 131 cases were rated good in general speech ability and 119 were rated poor. The results are found in Table 54.

The variances of the scores of the mild and severe cases are heterogeneous. When a modified *t* is applied the significance level is .001. Since the differences between means in terms of two different external criteria are highly significant, they may be taken as evidence for the validity of the test.

Replication of the Study

Since considerable use was made of this short test it was thought wise to replicate the study. Form I was administered to a second group of children with cerebral palsy. There were 114 subjects between the ages of 3 and 16 years in this group. They were from the states of Arizona, California, Colorado, Idaho, Kansas, New Mexico, Oregon, Utah and Washington. The result of replicating the study is presented in the following table.

The difference of 1.7 between the means of the two administrations of the test is not significant. The *p* value fails to attain the .05 level. Since the variances of the two sets of scores are homogeneous, and the means are not significantly different the second administration of the test verifies the result of the first administration.

TABLE 55
Replication of the Test of Ten Consonants

Administration	Mean	σ	diff	t	df	p
First	20.3	8.7				
Second	22.0	7.8	1.7	1.83	445	.10

Order of Item Difficulty

The order of difficulty of the items in the three positions in words is not the same. Table 56 indicates the different orders of difficulty from most to least for children with cerebral palsy.

It will be noted that for these children the voiced consonant ð and the voiceless sound ⊖ are among the most difficult. The s and z consonants are moderately difficult and the l and r sounds appear to be easier for these children to articulate. The order of difficulty according to the tally of the lists reported in the literature and the orders of difficulty for children with cerebral palsy agree in some respects but fail in others. The s and z consonants were listed in the literature as difficult and the r and l sounds as easiest. But the ∂ and ⊖ sounds are not as high on this list as they are for children with cerebral palsy. The t sound is comparable except for the final position. The placement of d and t on the lists are not consistent. The mean percent of difficulty of the items of the test for cerebral palsied children is 69, the range is 48 to 87. In view of the fact that a desirable range would be about 15% to 90% this range is somewhat restricted.

TABLE 56
Order of Difficulty of Items in the D.O.I. Test of Ten Consonants in Three Positions Using Cerebral Palsied Children

Initial	Medial	Final
ð	ð	z
⊖	ʃ	t
z	⊖	s
s	z	⊖
ʃ	s	tʃ
dʒ	dʒ	ð
r	tʃ	dʒ
tʃ	t	r
l	r	ʃ
t	l	l

Discriminating Power of the Items

An item has discriminating power if individuals who respond

correctly to it, on the average, are superior in general achievement to subjects who respond incorrectly. If all testees did equally well on the item it would lack discriminating power. This factor is measured by the correlation of the scores on the item with the scores of the test as a whole, and it is considered to be acceptable if the correlations are relatively high.

The correlation indicating discriminating power were found to be relatively high. The mean is .74 and the range is from .56 to .89.

Uniqueness of the Items

The uniqueness of an item means that two items do not duplicate the same function in a test. If the intercorrelations of items are high, item uniqueness is not present. The intercorrelations should be relatively low. The phi coefficient may be used to determine uniqueness.

The average intercorrelation is .30 and the range is from .13 to .59. Thus the values for uniqueness of items are quite low and contrast with a mean of .74 for their discriminating power. There is only a small overlap between the ranges, that for the discriminating power being .56 to .89. This test then meets fairly well the criteria of low intercorrelations for uniqueness and high correlations for discriminating power.

SUMMARY

A test of ten difficult consonants devised by Dale O. Irwin for use with mentally retarded children was administered to 333 children with cerebral palsy. The purpose was to standardize this test on cerebral palsied children for use with this type of child. The selection of the ten sounds was based on a tally of lists of difficult consonants reported in the literature. The sounds were s, z, $d\mathwith{3}$, $t\int$, Θ, $\int$, ∂, r, t, and $\mathl$. They were placed in the initial, medial and final positions in words. In standardizing the test on children with cerebral palsy an attempt was made to meet several criteria: (1) observer reliability, (2) test reliability, (3) validity of the test by means of the method of extreme groups, (4) verification by replication, (5) difficulty of the items, (6) their discriminating power and (7) their uniqueness.

Observer reliability was established using one hundred tape records of the articulation of twenty-two children with cerebral palsy and fifty-seven records of ten mentally retarded children. The mean percent of agreements by two observers was 95. Test reliability was calculated in three ways. A Kuder-Richardson formula yielded indices of internal consistency of .86 for initial consonants, .87 for medials and .86 for finals. A test-retest coefficient was .87. This is a measure of temporal stability. The coefficient of correlation between parallel forms was .85. These coefficients are quite similar. Validity was determined by the method of extreme groups. When the mean scores of children with cerebral palsy were diagnosed as mild and severe the difference between the mean articulation scores of the groups was significant at the .001 level. When therapists rated the children's general language ability as good or poor, the difference between the means also was significant at the .001 level. A replication of the test with a group of children from the western part of the country yielded a correlation of .85. There was no significant difference between the means, and the variances were homogeneous. The average percent of difficulty of the consonants was 69, the range was from 48 to 87. This range is too restricted. The mean discriminating power of the items is indicated by an r of .74, the range being from .56 to .89. The uniqueness of the items varies from .13 to .59 with a mean of .39. This mean is in contrast to that of .74 for discriminating power. Thus the relationship between these two aspects of the test is satisfactory.

Chapter 30

Correct Articulation of Ten Difficult Consonants by Children with Cerebral Palsy

THIS INVESTIGATION is concerned with the correct status of articulation of a set of ten difficult consonants by children with cerebral palsy. The test is found in Chart 10 of the Appendix.

The aims of the study are to determine (1) if there are sex differences in the scores, (2) what the relation is to chronological and mental ages, (3) the relation to the IQ, (4) the effect of the position of consonants in words, (5) if there are differences between right and left hemiplegics, (6) relation to medical diagnosis and (7) the relation to the extent of involvement.

PROCEDURE

The selection of the ten consonants was based on a tally of sounds common to lists of difficult sounds for several populations as they were reported in the literature. The consonants were used in words in the initial, medial and final positions. The test was constructed by Dale O. Irwin. The child was seated before a microphone in a quiet examining room and a few minutes were devoted to putting him at ease. The list of words then was read to him and he was instructed to repeat them one by one. The child's verbal responses were recorded on tape.

RESULTS

The Effect of Sex

There is no significant difference between the scores of the boys and girls. The mean for the boys is 20.2 with a standard deviation of 8.6. For the girls the mean is 20.3 and the standard deviation is 8.3. The means are equal and the variances are homogeneous.

Relation to Chronological Age, Mental Age and IQ

The correlation of the articulation scores and chronological age

142

is .04, with mental age it is −.03, and with the IQ it is .16. It is interesting to find that with cerebral palsied children the correlations of chronological age, mental age and IQ with the articulation of a set of difficult consonants yield correlations too low for predictive purposes.

It was noted that 79% of the IQs were below 90 and that 44% were below 70.

The Effect of Position

The means and standard deviations for the consonants in the initial, medial and final positions in words are 7.4 ± 3.0, 6.9 ± 3.1 and 6.2 ± 3.1.

It will be observed that the standard deviations are the same; the variances of the three groups are homogeneous. In view of the fact that in previous studies the analysis of variance always showed that the differences among the means of position proved to be significant, an analysis of variance of the above data was not run but tests of the differences among the means were determined. It was found that all differences were significant.

Relation to Right and Left Hemiplegia

Forty-nine children were available for this analysis. The value for right hemiplegics was 21.3 ± 9.0 and for left it was 21.5 ± 9.9.

By inspection the means are practically identical and the variances are homogeneous. Thus there does not appear to be any difference between these groups in their ability to phonate difficult consonants. A similar result was reported in the chapter on the status of final double consonant blends. These are unexpected findings as was earlier pointed out.

Relation to Medical Diagnosis

In this section a comparison will be made of the articulatory status of 187 spastics and 77 athetoids and tension athetoids. The means and standard deviations are spastics 22.3 ± 7.7, athetoids 16.8 ± 9.4.

Since the variances are heterogeneous a Modified Cochran-Cox t-test was applied to the data. The difference of 5.5 was significant at the .001 level. Thus on difficult consonants the two groups differ both in regard to the means and to the variances. This is a different finding from that with initial double consonant blends and with final double consonant blends. In both of these analyses the means and variances are alike. But with this set of consonants the spastics do better than the athetoids.

Relation to Extent of Involvement

In this sample there were available 189 quadriplegics, 53 hemiplegics and 48 paraplegics. The mean of the paraplegics exceeds that of the hemiplegics which in turn exceeds that of the quadriplegics. The values are 23.4, 21.8 and 18.9. The variances of the three groups are homogeneous. T-tests were applied to the differences among the means. The differences between the quadriplegics and hemiplegics, and between the quadriplegics and paraplegics, are significant at the .05 and .001 levels, but the difference between the means of the hemiplegics and paraplegics is not significant. The finding that the quadriplegics are inferior to the other two groups is consistent with results of previous studies.

SUMMARY

This study describes and analyzes the correct status of ten difficult consonants in the speech of 333 children with cerebral palsy from 3 to 16 years of age. The list of consonants was constructed by Dale O. Irwin and was based on a tally of sounds common to lists of difficult consonants for several populations as reported in the literature. The aims of the study were to determine (1) if there are sex differences in the scores, (2) what the relation is to chronological and mental ages and the IQ, (3) the effect of position of consonants in words, (4) if there are differences between right and left hemiplegics and (5) the relation to the medical diagnosis and the extent of involvement.

The following results were found: there was no significant difference between the scores of boys and girls. The means were alike and the variances were homogeneous. The scores of the ten consonants correlated .04 with chronological age. They correlated −.03 with mental age, and .16 with the IQ. The children did best with initial consonants. Medial and final consonants ranked below initials in that order. The differences among the means were all significant and the variances were homogeneous. The means of right and left hemiplegics were identical and the variances were homogeneous. The mean differences between the quadriplegics and hemiplegics, and between the quadriplegics and paraplegics, were such that the null hypothesis could be rejected, but the difference between the means of the hemiplegics and paraplegics was not significant.

Chapter 31

Comparison of Articulation Scores of Cerebral Palsied and Mentally Retarded Children

~~~~~~

THIS CHAPTER PRESENTS a comparison of the articulation of ten difficult consonants by cerebral palsied and mentally retarded children. The investigation is concerned with the following relationships: (1) a comparison of correct articulation scores of children with cerebral palsy with an IQ range of 25 to 50 with scores of retarded non–brain-damaged children with the same IQ range; (2) a similar comparison of the scores of the two groups with an IQ range of 51 to 80; (3) a comparison of cerebral palsied children with IQs of 91 to 110 with retarded children with IQs of 51 to 80; (4) a comparison of correct scores by cerebral palsied children with IQ range of 91 to 110 with the scores of non–cerebral-palsied children with the same IQ range; (5) a comparison of substitution errors of cerebral palsied children and retarded children with an IQ range of 25 to 50; (6) a similar comparison of substitution errors of two groups with the IQ range of 51 to 80; (7) a comparison of omission errors of the two groups with an IQ range of 25 to 50; and (8) a similar comparison of omissions by two groups with an IQ range of 51 to 80.

PROCEDURE

From a pool of cerebral palsied children from twenty-one states in New England, the Deep South and the Midwest, three groups were drawn. In the 25 to 50 IQ range there were twenty-four children, in the 51 to 80 IQ range there were fifty-eight cases, and in the mentally normal cerebral-palsied group (IQ between 91 and 110) there were twenty-six children. The mentally retarded groups each included forty-one children in the IQ ranges of 25 to 50 and 51 to 80. These two groups were diagnosed as being without brain damage. In addition a group of forty-one otherwise

146

normal children with IQ ranges of 91 to 110 was included in the study. These three groups were from the public schools of Cedar Rapids, Iowa. They were matched on chronological age and economic status. The mean chronological age of the trainable mentally retarded children was 10 years, 5 months. The mean of the educable mentally retarded was 9 years, 9 months. The mean chronological age for the children with cerebral palsy was 9 years, 4 months.

The test used in this study consisted of ten consonants based on a tally of sounds common to lists of difficult sounds for several populations of children reported in the literature.

RESULTS

Table 57 represents the correct articulation scores of the ten consonants of the several groups of children. The first section reveals that the mean for the cerebral palsied children with IQs of 25 to 50 is 16.0, while the mean for the retarded of the same IQ range is 21.2. The difference between the means in favor of the retarded group is significant at the .01 level. When the means of the two groups with IQs of 51 to 80 are compared, again the retarded exceed the children with cerebral palsy. The significance level is .05.

TABLE 57

Ten Difficult Consonants Comparison of Two Groups of Cerebral Palsied, Retarded and Normal Children on Articulation Scores

	Correct Scores				
	IQ 25 to 50				
	Mean	*diff*	*t*	*df*	*p*
Cerebral Palsied	16.0				
Retarded	21.2	5.2	2.84	63	.01
	IQ 51 to 80				
Cerebral Palsied	21.1				
Retarded	25.1	4.0	2.15	97	.05
	CP 91 to 110, Retarded 51 to 80				
Cerebral Palsied	24.7				
Retarded	25.1	0.4	0.25	65	.80
	CP 91 to 110, Normal 91 to 110				
Cerebral Palsied	24.7				
Non–Cerebral Palsied	29.7	5.0	5.89	65	.001

Whenever variances were heterogeneous the Cochran-Cox Modified t was applied.

The third section of the table compares the articulation of children with cerebral palsy with IQs in the normal range (91 to 110) with the articulation of retarded children with IQs of 51 to 80. It is seen that the two means when rounded are the same and that the difference is at the .80 level. The children with cerebral palsy with normal intelligence thus do no better than retarded children with the IQ range of 51 to 80.

The last section of the table compares the articulation of the ten consonants by cerebral palsied children of normal intelligence with that of normal children (IQ 91 to 110). The children with cerebral palsy are seen to be inferior to the non–cerebral-palsied children. The difference of 5.0 between the means is significant at the .001 level.

The data in Table 57 then suggest that retarded children do better in the correct articulation of the ten most difficult sounds than children with cerebral palsy of the same intelligence range.

Table 58 gives data comparing the two IQ groups of retarded and cerebral palsied children on errors of substitution and omission.

The first section compares the two IQ groups with the range of 25 to 50. It indicates that children with cerebral palsy make significantly more substitution errors than the retarded children,

TABLE 58

Comparison of Two Groups of Cerebral Palsied and Retarded Children on Articulation Errors

		Substitutions			
		IQ 25 to 50			
	Mean	*diff*	*t*	*df*	*p*
Cerebral Palsied	7.3				
Retarded	3.1	4.2	4.29	63	.001
		IQ 51 to 80			
Cerebral Palsied	4.2				
Retarded	3.6	0.6	0.74	97	.50
		IQ 25 to 50			
Cerebral Palsied	5.8				
Retarded	5.4	0.4	0.49	63	.60
		IQ 51 to 80			
Cerebral Palsied	3.3				
Retarded	1.2	2.1	0.37	97	.70

Whenever variances were heterogeneous the Cochran-Cox Modified t was applied.

but that the groups in the 51 to 80 IQ range are alike. When the means are rounded the values are alike. The second half of the table indicates that in regard to omission the differences are not significant.

SUMMARY

When retarded and cerebral palsied children with IQs of 25 to 50 are compared for their ability to articulate ten difficult consonant sounds, the retarded group does better significantly than the cerebral palsied group. A similar result obtains for the two groups whose IQ range is 51 to 80. When children with cerebral palsy whose IQ range is 91 to 110 are compared with retarded children with a range from 51 to 80, the means of the two groups are not significantly different. When cerebral palsied children with an IQ range of 91 to 110 are compared with non–cerebral-palsied children of the same range, the cerebral palsied children are inferior. The difference between the means is significant at the .001 level. In regard to substitutions, cerebral palsied children with IQs 25 to 50 make more errors than retarded children of the same intelligence level. The two groups in the IQ range of 51 to 80 make about the same mean number of substitution errors. In regard to omissions, for both the IQ ranges of 25 to 50 and of 51 to 80, the mean differences between the two groups of children are not significant.

DISCUSSION

As far as the articulation of difficult consonants is concerned, from this analysis there appears to be experimental evidence that cerebral palsy in addition to mental retardation may be a real factor. What the amount of influence of this factor might be is at present speculative. However, in another study it was found that correct articulation scores of cerebral palsy correlated .53 with oral muscular difficulties. The corresponding coefficient of determination r^2 is 28. This means that about 28% of the variances of the two factors overlap. If this value is at all reliable, it might be inferred that the oral paralyses in cerebral palsied children are penalizing these children in addition to their mental retardation in an amount of about 25%. This value although suggestive is hypothetical. The problem of quantifying the oral paralytic factor in relation to faulty articulation needs further investigation.

Chapter 32

A Second Comparative Study of Articulation of Cerebral Palsied and Mentally Retarded Children

IN THE PRECEEDING CHAPTER a comparison was made of the articulation scores of cerebral palsied and mentally retarded children. In that study a test consisting of ten difficult consonants was used. It was found that trainable mentally retarded children—that is, those with IQs in the range of 25 to 50—made a significantly higher mean articulation score than cerebral palsied children in the same IQ range. Also it was found that educable mentally retarded children—that is, those in the IQ range of 51 to 80—did better on the test than cerebral palsied children in this range. In view of the fact that about 80% of children with cerebral palsy had IQ scores below normal the study provided at least tentative evidence that the affliction of cerebral palsy as such is a factor in addition to the mental retardation of these children.

The aim of the present investigation is to learn if this hypothesis holds for a more complete set of vowel and consonant phonemes employing the Integrated Articulation Test. The analysis will be made in two parts. First the means and standard deviations of the cerebral palsied cases will be compared with mentally retarded children, disregarding the IQ range. This will be done in terms of correct articulation and in terms of substitution and omission errors. The second part of the study will deal with the two types of children each divided into two subgroups. The division again will be on the basis of the IQ range. That is, the articulation of cerebral palsied children in the IQ range of 25 to 50 will be compared with mentally retarded children in the same range, and cerebral palsied children with IQs between 51 and 80 will be compared with mentally retarded children in this range. Another aim of the study will be to determine the relative frequency of

151

omission and substitution errors in the articulation of cerebral palsied children and also of mentally retarded children.

PROCEDURE

There were 162 mentally retarded children between three and sixteen years inclusive from the five states of California, Idaho, Michigan, Nebraska and Wyoming. Also there were 265 children with cerebral palsy of the same range from fifteen states of California, Idaho, Illinois, Indiana, Iowa, Kansas, Kentucky, Michigan, Montana, Nebraska, Nevada, Ohio, West Virginia, Wisconsin and Wyoming.

RESULTS

Differences Between Cerebral Palsied and Mentally Retarded Children

The means and standard deviations of the group of 265 children with cerebral palsy and the 162 mentally retarded children for correct articulation scores and for the two more prominent types of articulation errors, namely substitutions and omissions, have been calculated. They are found in Table 59.

Table 59 provides several items of information about the two types of children. The first concerns the relative ability of the two groups to articulate correctly. The average mentally retarded child achieves a higher mean correct score than the cerebral palsied child. The mean for the cerebral palsied children is 64.0, while that for the mentally retarded children is 75.1. The variances of the two sets of scores, as indicated by the standard deviations, are homogeneous. The table also reveals that the cerebral palsied subjects make more substitution and omission errors than the mentally retarded children. Also the standard deviations indicate that variances of the error distributions are heterogeneous.

The means of the table have been subjected to tests of significance. An assumption for the application of an analysis of variance to several populations is that the variance of the measures is the same. Since the variances over the table are heterogeneous, t-tests have been applied. The probability values are presented in Table 59.

TABLE 59

t Values of Differences of Means Between Cerebral Palsied and Mentally Retarded Children on Correct Articulation Scores, Substitutions and Omissions

	M	diff	t	df	p
		Correct Scores			
Cerebral Palsied	64.0	21.1			
Mentally Retarded	75.1	22.1	11.1	5.16	425	.001
		Substitutions			
Cerebral Palsied	81.0	7.3			
Mentally Retarded	47.0	4.4	34.0	53.00	425	.001
		Omissions			
Cerebral Palsied	86.3	7.1			
Mentally Retarded	67.0	6.0	19.3	27.40	425	.001

For correct scores t-tests yield a probability value which lies at the .001 level providing evidence of the superiority of articulatory ability of mentally retarded children over children with cerebral palsy.

Frequency of Substitutions and Omissions

Table 59 provides another item of information. This concerns the frequency of substitution and omission errors. In the case of both the mentally retarded and the cerebral palsied child the mean for omissions exceeds that for substitutions. For both cerebral palsied and mentally retarded children, it is seen that omissions significantly exceed substitutions. The null hypothesis may be rejected at the .001 level.

The results shown in Table 59 accordingly may be taken as a verification of the hypothesis that the affliction of cerebral palsy as such is a factor in addition to the mental retardation of these children.

SUMMARY AND CONCLUSION

This study is an attempt to answer two questions: (1) is the affliction of cerebral palsy a factor in addition to mental retardation in the speech of the cerebral palsied child and (2) what is the relative frequency of substitution and omission errors in the articulation of cerebral palsied children and also of mentally retarded children. There were 162 mentally retarded children from 3 to 16 years of age inclusive from five states, and 265 cerebral palsied children of the same age range from fifteen states. The children were given an articulation test consisting of eighty-seven words involving thirty-five vowels and consonants.

The date compiled in this investigation constitute a vertification of the hypothesis derived from an earlier study that cerebral palsy as such is a factor in addition to the mental retardation in the speech of cerebral palsied children. This is evidenced by the fact that mentally retarded children make better scores on the articulation test than cerebral palsied children. The second aim was to learn if omissions by cerebral palsied and mentally retarded children exceed substitutions. The analysis showed that the difference, in both groups of children, was of a size sufficient to reject the null hypothesis. This is the reverse of the finding with normal children whose substitution errors exceed omissions.

Chapter 33

The Relation of a Short to a Long Consonant Test

PROCEDURE

SHORT AND LONG consonant articulation tests were administered to 139 handicapped children who were patients in the Institute of Logopedics at Wichita, Kansas. The purpose of the study was to determine the degree of correlation between the two tests. A short test frequently may be used when economy of time and cost are imperative.

Description of the Tests

The short consonant test was designed for the purpose of quick evaluation of a subject's phonetic ability. It was constructed using ten difficult consonants which were common to lists of the most difficult sounds reported in the literature for various populations. Each consonant is presented in the initial, medial and final positions in words. The test was standardized for use with cerebral palsied children. Item analyses were done and the reliability and validity of the test were established. Two forms of the test are charted in the Appendix.

The long test used in this study consisted of the consonant parts of a series of tests for use with cerebral palsied and mentally retarded children. The items were selected by means of an analysis involving the difficulty of the items, their discriminating power and their uniqueness. Reliability and validity of the longer tests were established satisfactorily. There are thirty items in the short test and sixty-seven in the long test.

RESULTS

The mean score for the test with ten difficult consonants was 19.4. The standard deviation was 9.1. This is comparable to a mean of 20.3 ± 8.7 obtained in a previous study. This is further indication of the reliability of the short test. The mean for the longer test was 51.4 and the standard deviation was 17.6.

When the scores of the two tests were correlated the coefficient was found to be .90. The coefficient of determination r^2 is .81 and the forecasting efficiency was 56%. Thus the short test predicts results of the long test with reasonable efficiency. Whenever economy of cost and time dictate it, the short test of difficult consonants may be used in place of the longer instrument. Moreover it may be used with a considerable degree of reliability to evaluate the consonantal ability of a mixed population of children.

A summary of the results of the various analyses of articulation will be found in the final chapter. It is pertinent at this point, however, to emphasize that these analyses define and elaborate articulation as an operational construct. The meaning of articulation is determined and bound up in the instructions, procedural rules, tests and operations which have been utilized in its investigation and in the results which have been obtained. Having in this manner developed a construct of articulation, it now may enter into and become a part of the broader constitutive type of definition or construct of communication.

This concludes the analyses of articulation problems of cerebral palsied and mentally retarded children.

PART II
SOUND DISCRIMINATION

The initial chapter presented reasons why the function of sound discrimination is basic to the art of communication. It was indicated that discrimination is the response in the communicative situation. Its peculiar function in the situation, however, is dual. Sound discrimination is not only a response but its expression becomes a stimulating factor in the situation. A discrimination is a response and it is a stimulus. It should be illuminating to learn the abilities and deficiencies of cerebral palsied and mentally retarded children in the sound discrimination situation.

It should be reiterated that the variable of sound discrimination as well as each of the remaining variables may be viewed as an operational definition which illuminates the constitutive construct of communication.

Chapter 34

A Test of Sound Discrimination

SIX STUDIES on sound discrimination by cerebral palsied and mentally retarded children were completed. Tests appropriate to this type of child were constructed and administered to about 660 children. The data were analyzed and are presented here.

PROCEDURE AND RESULTS
Form A, Part I

This is a second project on the construction of tests for use with children with cerebral palsy. The first project was concerned with articulation. The present purpose is to standardize two equivalent tests, Forms A and B, which may be used to investigate the ability of these children to discriminate speech sounds. Part I of Form A will be devoted to a description of the subjects used in this part of the project, to a consideration of sex and geographical differences, to the question of the reliability of the observations and to an analysis of the items of Form A. It will be noted that 61% of the children have a mental status of an IQ of 90 and less, that 33% have IQs less than 70.

Sex and Geographical Differences

In order to find if there were differences between the mean scores of boys and girls in two geographical regions, a simple analysis of variance was done. The geographical regions consisted of states in the Southwest and in the East. Table 60 gives the means and standard deviations of the four groups.

Inspection of the standard deviations of the four groups reveals that the variances are fairly homogeneous. An analysis of

Note: This study was conducted and written with the collaboration of Paul J. Jensen.

TABLE 60
Means and Standard Deviations of Boys and Girls in Two Geographical Regions

	Southwest			East		
	N	M	σ	N	M	σ
Boys	42	16.3	5.5	39	16.9	5.0
Girls	38	15.7	6.1	34	17.2	5.1

variance was applied to determine if the central tendencies are significantly different. Since the analysis of variance yielded an F ratio of less than one, the null hypothesis may be accepted. In other words there are no sex differences and no geographical differences. Consequently the scores of boys and girls in the two geographical regions may be considered to belong to the same population and subsequent analyses of the data may be based on the entire sample of scores. This result is similar to that found with articulation.

Reliability of the Observer

Two observers read the taped responses of sixty-five children with speech difficulties. Both Forms A and B of the sound discrimination tests were administered to the children. Twenty-nine were cerebral palsied children, and twenty were articulatory cases. There were five mentally retarded children and eleven aphasic children. The percentages of agreement of the two observers listening independently amounted to 96%. This is an adequate observer reliability value, but it also means that a 4% error exists in the data.

Item Analysis

The project was carried out in several stages. The first step was to assemble a pool of items (paired words). This was done by consulting the literature on sound discrimination, *Webster's Unabridged Dictionary*, testbooks on phonetics and words included a number of articulation tests. The pool of items consisted of 135 paired words. The next stage was to reduce the pool to one hundred words. This was done in consultation with a speech pathologist experienced in the speech problems of cerebral palsied children.* These items then were divided into two groups

*Appreciation is expressed to Dr. Ralph Schwartz, member of the staff of the Institute of Logopedics.

of fifty each for the eventual construction of two equivalent tests which will be designated as Form A and Form B. The construction and standardization of Form A was accomplished in two further stages. The fifty-item test was administered in a preliminary tryout to a group of eighty-six cerebral palsied children in six rehabilitation centers in Kansas, Oklahoma and Texas. An item analysis was then made and on this basis the number of test items was further reduced to twenty-five. It was then taken out for a final administration with a second sample of 153 children in the states of Arizona, California, Delaware, Indiana, Kansas, Missouri, New Jersey, New Mexico, New York, Tennessee and Texas. The reliability and validity of the final form was determined on the scores of the second sample. These two matters will be treated in Part II of this study.

The item analysis was made on the basis of three criteria: (1) the discriminating power of each item and that of uniqueness using the cutting point of $r = .50$, and then noting if the percent of difficulty of the item fell within the range of 20 to 85. Thus the item ("pig-big") had a discriminating power of $r = .81$ and a uniqueness value of $r = .22$. Its percent of difficulty was 73, which is within the ideal range. These criterion values make this item eligible for the final form. The item ("habitat-habitant") has a value of $r = .63$ for discriminating power, of $r = .04$ for uniqueness, and a percent of difficulty of 57. Occasionally the selection rule was violated as in the case of ("chip-ship") for which the r for discriminating power was low. This was compensated by an r of .05 for uniqueness. Moreover, speech therapists report that children often need help with the ("ch-sh") pair.

On the basis of this analysis the items were reassembled into the final form of Test A. The new form is found in Table 61. In addition to the twenty-five items of the new form, five foils in parentheses are included. The purpose of the foils is to enable the tester to check if the testee is attending properly to the task.

The table reveals that the mean discriminating power of the 25 items of the final form is $r = .65$, with a range of .11 to .87. For uniqueness the mean is $r = .19$ and the range is .01 to .28. The mean for item difficulty is 68% with a range from 36% to 80%. On

TABLE 61
Final Form A
Sound Discrimination Test for Use with Cerebral Palsied Children

Item	Discrim. Power r	Mean Uniqueness	Diff. %
1. tin-thin	60	21	80
2. late-date	73	25	78
3. pig-big	81	22	73
4. (gun-gun)			
5. test-text	65	19	71
6. bud-bug	51	27	70
7. chip-ship	11	01	36
8. habitat-habitant	63	04	57
9. sop-shop	79	20	67
10. conical-comical	45	11	58
11. (hoe-hoe)			
12. beats-beads	76	22	65
13. cytology-psychology	63	26	64
14. class-clasp	62	13	72
15. mush-much	57	12	74
16. patriarch-matriarch	81	27	69
17. (peach-peach)			
18. wear-where	87	26	57
19. biscuit-brisket	79	28	69
20. foal-stole	59	14	80
21. pass-path	33	03	41
22. convergent-conversant	76	21	77
23. falls-false	62	21	76
24. (at-at)			
25. refracted-retracted	79	25	73
26. coke-cope	79	26	76
27. carrion-Marion	76	25	73
28. (far-far)			
29. frisking-whisking	60	20	74
30. thigh-sigh	77	13	76
Mean r = .65		r = .19	% = .63
Range = .11–.87		.01–.28	36–80

the whole, the test items meet the three criteria of discriminating power, uniqueness and difficulty. The inclusion of item 7 with a discriminating power of .11 extends the range too far below the cutting value of .50. Otherwise the range is satisfactory.

Summary

Neither sex nor geographical differences were present. Observer reliability was quite satisfactory, the percent of agreement between two observers was 96. This means that there is a 4% error in the data. The selection of items was based on a threefold analysis: (1) discriminating power of the items, (2) their uniqueness and (3) the percent of difficulty of the items. Twenty-five of the fifty items met these criteria and were incorporated in the final edition of Form A.

Form A, Part II

Part II is concerned specifically with the reliability and validity of the sound discrimination test for cerebral palsied children and deals with several additional problems. They are the administration of the test, a comparison of the sound discrimination abilities of spastics and athetoids, of quadriplegics, hemiplegics and paraplegics. It includes also an analysis of the scores in the initial, medial and final positions in the test words, and a statement of the effect of chronological age, mental age and IQ on the scores.

In Part I it was pointed out that neither sex nor geographical effects on the scores were present and that consequently the subjects of these samples belong to the same population. Therefore the present analysis may be made on the group as a whole. The mean sound discrimination score of the 153 children is 16.6 with a standard deviation of 5.7. The maximum score on the test is 25.0.

Reliability of Form A

The reliability of the test was determined by means of a Kuder-Richardson formula. The coefficient of reliability derived by the formula was $r = .87$.*

A further indication of the reliability of the test is afforded by an analysis of variance in which the two sexes and the two geographical areas are entered. The result, reported in Part I, showed no significant differences among the means. Consequently each group mean verifies the other group means. This is another demonstration of the internal consistency or of the reliability of the test.

---

*Although the maximum score on Form A is 25, the coefficient of reliability was calculated by including the scores on five foils.

Validity of Form A

The reliability of a test is based on an internal criterion. The validity of a test is in terms of an external criterion. The external criterion may be chronological or mental age or teacher's or therapist's rating.

The first analysis will be of the chronological age progression of the sound discrimination scores. For this purpose the age range of 6 to 17 years was divided into six age levels. An age level consists of a two-year period. The mean sound discrimination scores varied from 13.8 ± 5.0 at the first age level of 6 years, to 18.9 ± 5.4 at 16 years.

The variances are homogeneous, consequently it was possible to apply an F test to the means. The analysis of variance yielded an F of 5.48, with df = 5 and 145, p = .001. Thus the trend of the scores with chronological age was significant. Since chronological age is an external criterion, the significant age trend may be taken as evidence of the validity of Form A.

A similar approach to the validity of the test may be made by an examination of the trend of mental age scores. In this case the levels composed of two-year periods have had to be reduced to four because of the scarcity of cases in the levels above 9 to 10. That is, the cases of these older levels were included in the 9 to 10 level. The scores varied with 12.8 ± 5.8 at the 3 to 4 year level to 21.3 ± 3.0 at the 9 to 16 mental age level.

An analysis of variance yielded an F of 10.7, df = 3 and 88, p = .001, indicating a significant trend in the scores with mental age of Form A.

Another analysis which bears on the validity of the test deals with the ratings of the general language ability and speech intelligibility of the children. The means and standard deviations of the therapists' ratings of very good, good, medium, poor and very poor progressed from 15.9 ± 5.8 for very poor to 18.5 ± 5.0 for very good.

An analysis of variance was done on the values of the table with df (4,141). F = 2.41, p = .05. The differences among the means were significant at the .05 level. These results afford added evidence for the validity of the test.

Relation to Medical Diagnosis

An analysis was made of the scores of the children in terms of the medical diagnosis of mild, moderate and severe involvement. The values are 15.8 ± 6.7, 16.6 ± 5.5, and 16.9 ± 5.5.

Interestingly, the mean value for the mildly involved cases is somewhat less than the means of the moderate and severe. However, the differences among the means are not significant. $F = 1.48$, $df = 39$ and 55, and $p = 10\%$. The variances are homogeneous. Thus it is seen that the scores according to the medical diagnosis reveal no significant differences.

In summarizing these analyses according to the method of extreme groups, the progression of the scores according to both chronological and mental age affords evidence for the validity of Form A. The analysis of the groups rated by the speech therapist likewise is significant. The analysis based on the medical diagnosis, however, reveals no differences which are significant. In other words with degree of paralytic involvement, the three trends still are significant.

Up to this point in Part I and II of this report, a series of problems concerning the construction of a sound discrimination test for use with cerebral palsied children have been discussed, including an explanation of three criteria whereby an item analysis of a test may be made, and the selection by means of these criteria of a number of items based on a preliminary sample of children. A determination on a second sample also was made in order to establish observer reliability. Then, with a third sample of children several kinds of test reliability and validity were determined. Something now should be said concerning the manner of administering the test to the cerebral palsied child.

Instructions for Administering the Test

A number of conditions should be observed during the testing period. After the child is brought to a quiet examining room, he should be seated facing the examiner who sits with his face in a good light. Considerable effort should be made to put the child at ease. A few moments of conversation will usually help.

The child should be tested for hearing. This can be done by means of an audiometer if it is available. A sweep of about 10 to

15 decibels at frequencies of 500, 1000, 2000 and 4000 usually is sufficient to establish if the child hears adequately. Also the child may be asked to repeat a few spondaic words such as "birthday," "baseball," "airplane," "cowboy," "hotdog" and "oatmeal." A few questions and a direction or two also will satisfy the therapist that the child responds. Examples may be, How many legs does a man have? Does a cow eat hay or stones? Give the pencil to me. Put the pencil on the table.

After the tester is satisfied that the child has adequate hearing, the sound discrimination test may be administered. Form A of the test is given in Chart 12 (see Appendix). Instructions to the child are given in the heading. They are as follows: "I am going to say two words. Sometimes the words will sound the same. Then you say 'same.' Sometimes parts of the words will be the same but other parts will sound different. Then you say 'different.' Let's try some words. 'Ma-pa.' Do they sound the same or do they sound different?" Other items are "boy-toy," "noon-moon," "leave-leash." After this short practice session the thirty items of the test should be given. The examiner should speak slowly and clearly at an ordinary conversational level, or louder if the situation demands it. Care should be taken to separate the two words of a pair with a slight pause. If the therapist suspects that the child is a lip-reader, he can say the words behind his hand. When saying the pair, the voice should be kept even on both words. If the voice is kept up on the first word, it should be kept up on the second, otherwise an extraneous cue might be given to the subject.

Some children will do better if required to give a "yes" or "no" response. Sometimes a child will not be able to respond verbally. In this case an affirmative nod or negative shake of the head will suffice. With younger children and those with low mental ages, a difficulty may be encountered because some of the children may not be mature enough to understand the difference in the meaning of "same" and "different." The following device may then be used. Ask if the sounds are the same. If he replies with "same," then ask if the sounds are different. Sometimes the child may say "same" in both cases, or he may say "different" in both cases. The record sheet should be checked in the correct and error column but the item is counted as an error. This will give a cue that the child does not understand the task. The method should be continued with as many pairs as is necessary for the examiner to be satisfied that the child cannot be used as a subject.

Some children will exhibit perseveration in their responses. This may take the form of repeating the word "same" or the word "different" throughout a portion of the list. Or the child may echo the last part of the tester's question. Thus if the last word in the question is "same" or if it is "different," the child may echo the word "same" or the word "different" consistently. The situation may be handled by reversing the terms and asking, Are they different or the same? If there is echolalia the child will respond consistently. A check on how well the child is attending is afforded by five foils throughout the list. They are included in parentheses. If more foils are needed the examiner may insert them at random as the test proceeds. The responses to the foils are not included in the final score.

Attention is called to several blank spaces at the bottom of the test form.

Having discussed the details of administering the test, there remains the task of evaluating the relations of sound discrimination scores to several other variables. These concern the relation of test scores to chronological age, mental age and IQ, the effect of the position of sounds in words, the effect of spasticity and athetosis, and the effect of the extent of paralysis.

Relation of Test Scores to Chronological Age, Mental Age and IQ

The correlations of Form A scores with chronological age and with mental age are in the neighborhood of $r = .50$, while the correlation with IQ is .33. The coefficients of correlation may be evaluated in several ways. All three are significant at the 1% level. Another approach is by means of the coefficient of determination which is r^2. These values indicate the proportion of the variance of the scores which is accounted for by the variance of the correlated factor. In order, the coefficients of forecasting efficiency are 15, 14 and 6.

Effect of Position in Words

In order to determine if the effect of the position of the sound in the word is significant, the means and standard deviations were calculated. Since the N for the sounds in the middle position was small, its mean was omitted from the calculation. Those for the initial and final positions were used. The values are 9.1 ± 2.9 and 5.7 ± 2.8. The variances are homogeneous.

The difference of 3.4 between the means of the two positions is highly significant. This indicates that cerebral palsied children have greater difficulty in discriminating sounds in the final position than in the initial position. This result is consistent with what was found in the articulation of sounds by cerebral palsied children. The final sounds in words are more difficult for these children than initials.

Effect of Spasticity and Athetosis

With a test of the articulation of sounds, it was found that spastic children do better than athetoids. The present analysis is intended to find if they also do better in discriminating speech sounds. The mean for spastics is 16.4 ± 6.0 and for athetoids it is 17.0 ± 5.4, with df = 126, t = .50. The probability is at the .60 level.

It is evident that there is no significant difference between the sound discrimination means of spastics and athetoids. The variances were homogeneous. This result is in contrast to a significant difference found in the articulatory ability of these groups.

Effect of Extent of Paralysis

In the aforementioned study of articulation by cerebral palsied children, it was learned that quadriplegics make lower scores than hemiplegics and paraplegics and that the latter tend to make the highest scores. Here the aim is to find out if a similar situation is obtained with respect to sound discrimination. The means of the three groups are all 16.7 ± 5.6.

Thus the extent of physical paralysis has no effect on the sound discrimination of these children. This is in contrast to the finding on articulation.

Summary

The reliability of the test using a Kuder-Richardson formula is $r = .87$. Further confirming evidence of reliability is that the means of two widely different geographical samples are the same. Using the method of extreme groups for evaluating the validity of the test, the difference between the means of discrimination scores of extreme chronological age groups was found to be statistically significant. The difference between the means of discrimination scores of children rated good and poor in general language ability also was significant. The means of scores of children diagnosed medically as mild, moderate and severe were alike. The correlation of chronological age and sound discrimination scores was $r = .52$, of mental age and scores it was $r = .51$, and the correlation of IQ and sound discrimination scores was $r = .33$. The position of sounds in the words is a factor. The mean score of sounds in the initial position is significantly greater than in the final position. There is no significant difference between the mean scores of spastics and athetoids. The extent of physical paralysis has no effect on the means of the sound discriminations of quadriplegics, hemiplegics and paraplegics.

Chapter 35

A Parallel Test of Sound Discrimination

THIS REPORT CONCERNS the construction of a second test of sound discrimination for use with cerebral palsied children. It is designed as a parallel form (Form B) of a test previously reported which has been designated as Form A.

The report is organized in two parts. Part I includes a description of the subjects, a treatment of sex and geographical differences, and an item analysis. Part II discusses the reliability and validity of the test. It indicates also the relation of the test scores to age, IQ and type and extent of paralysis.

PROCEDURE AND RESULTS
Form B, Part I

Sex and Geographical Differences

The data were gathered in two different geographical areas, the North Central States and the Northwest States. In order to find out if boys and girls in these areas belong to the same population, an analysis of variance was done. The means and standard deviations are found in Table 62.

An analysis of variance revealed that the differences among the means are not significant. That is, there is no significant difference between the sexes and no difference between the regions. Consequently the scores of the groups may be considered to belong to the same population and subsequent analyses of the data may be

TABLE 62
Means and Standard Deviations of Sound Discrimination Scores (Form B)
of Boys and Girls in Two Geographical Areas

	Boys			Girls		
	N	M	σ	N	M	σ
North Central	80	18.7	5.4	71	19.7	3.9
Northwest	60	18.6	5.4	49	19.2	3.0

170

based on the entire sample of scores. The values of Table 62 are slightly higher than those of Table 60.

Item Analysis

The analysis of the items of Form B was done in terms of the usual criteria on data collected on a tryout group of 129 children. These were (1) the discriminating power of the items, (2) their uniqueness and (3) the difficulty of the items.

TABLE 63
Final Form B
Sound Discrimination Test for Use with Cerebral Palsied Children

	Item	Discriminating Power (r)	Mean Uniqueness (Φ)	Difficulty (%)
1.	leech-leash	61	17	65
2.	church-birch	56	16	83
3.	wrench-wench	64	12	71
4.	antecedent-antecedence	60	17	58
5.	(late-late)			
6.	defection-deflection	82	27	71
7.	retraction-detraction	74	28	75
8.	hydrolyte-hydrolize	71	28	86
9.	splashing-flashing	70	27	85
10.	(unearth-unearth)			
11.	tub-tug	62	17	74
12.	sloughs-sluice	76	27	81
13.	impellent-impeller	74	22	82
14.	hurting-herding	57	19	61
15.	denominate-renominate	68	26	85
16.	choke-joke	68	26	85
17.	(broom-broom)			
18.	fresh-flesh	69	25	85
19.	wreath-wreathe	70	30	83
20.	grieve-grief	76	26	78
21.	matter-madder	57	14	50
22.	(athlete-athlete)			
23.	boot-booed	73	33	81
24.	mobbing-mopping	72	30	79
25.	hydrochloric-hydrochlorid	68	15	72
26.	keyed-keen	73	30	80
27.	(poem-poem)			
28.	rheoscope-rheotrope	75	23	83
29.	oscillograph-oscillogram	72	13	81
30.	preceding-receding	72	29	81
		Mean r = .69 Range: .56–.82	Mean r = .23 Range: .12–.33	Mean % = 77 Range: 50–86

The selection of the twenty-five items for the final Form B was made by comparing the coefficients of correlation for discriminating power and of the uniqueness of each item using the cutting point of r = .50 and then noting if the percent of difficulty of the item fell within the range of 20% to 85%. The r for discriminating power should be greater than .50, while the phi coefficient for uniqueness should be less than .50. Thus the item ("leech-leash") had a discriminating power of .61, the uniqueness value was r = .17, and the percent of difficulty was 65. The criterion values of this item make it acceptable for inclusion in the final form of the test. Twenty-five items were selected in this manner. In addition five foils in parentheses were included. Their purpose is to enable the tester to check if the testee is attending properly to the task. The final form is found in Table 63.

The mean coefficient of correlation for discriminating power of the twenty-five items of Form B is r = .69. The range is .56 to .82. The mean phi coefficient for uniqueness is p = .23. The range is .12 to .33. Thus the mean value for discriminating power is quite high while that for uniqueness is low. The ranges do not overlap. The mean percent of difficulty is 77. This value is somewhat higher than the corresponding value of Form A indicating that Form B may be the easier of the two forms.

Summary

As in the case of Form A, neither sex nor geographical differences were present. On the basis of an item analysis including discriminating power, uniqueness and difficulty, twenty-five of the fifty-four items were incorporated into the final edition of Form B.

Form B, Part II

It was found above that neither sex nor geographical effects on the scores of Form B were present. Therefore the subjects of these samples belong to the same population and the following analyses may be made on the group as a whole.

Reliability of Form B

It was seen above that no significant differences were found among boys and girls in two geographical areas. This may be taken as evidence for the internal consistency of the data. Moreover when a Kuder-Richardson coefficient of reliability was applied, r = .88.

Forms A and B were both administered to a group of 260 cerebral palsied children in order to determine if the two forms are parallel. Parallel form reliability may be established if three criteria are met. These are (1) the means must not be significantly different, (2) the variances must be homogeneous and (3) the correlation between the two sets of scores must be substantial. The mean score for Form A is 19.0 ± 4.5. For Form B it is 19.1 ± 4.7. The correlation between the two forms is .90. It may therefore be inferred that the two forms of this test are equivalent.

Validity of Form B

The validity of the test was determined by the method of extreme groups. The concept of validity is based on the correspondence of a test with an external criterion. The external criterion may be chronological age, mental age or therapists' ratings. Age progression in the scores of a test means that there is a difference between extreme age groups. In other words the criterion of age progression implies the method of extreme groups for evaluating validity.

The age range of 6 to 17 years was divided into six age levels, each level consisting of a two-year period. The means of chronological age progressed from a score of 16.0 ± 4.7 for the youngest subjects to 21.8 ± 3.3 for the oldest age group. The standard deviations indicate that the variances are only slightly heterogeneous. Using a simple analysis of variance as a test for trends in means based on six independent samples, the F ratio was 3.57. With df (5, 248), p = .005 indicating there was a significant chronological age progression in the scores. Since age is an external criterion, this constitutes evidence of the validity of Form B. A similar result was found with Form A.

Another approach for determining the validity of the test is to evaluate the trend in the scores according to mental age. The trend in the scores with mental age varies from 16.2 ± 5.6 for the three- to four-year level to 23.5 ± 1.7 for the eleven to sixteen age group. An analysis of variance yielded an F of 14.36 which with p = .001 indicates a significant trend in the sound discrimination scores with mental age. It should be noted that the standard deviations decreased with age indicating heterogeneity of variance. However, the F ratio is so large that it is very doubtful that the significance of the progression is due to heterogeneity alone. In order to clarify the matter the difference between the means of the two extreme mental age groups was evaluated by the Cochran-Cox modified t. The Cochran-Cox modified t value was 2.81. Inasmuch as the observed *t* of 6.64 exceeds this value, the difference between the means of the extreme groups is significant and affords more evidence for the validity of the test.

Therapists' Ratings

An analysis was done using therapists' ratings of the speech intelligibility of the children and their overall language ability. The mean values range from 16.6 ± 5.5 for very poor to 20.8 ± 4.7, the very good rating. Variances were homogeneous.

It will be noted that the standard deviations are about the same. An analysis of variance reveals that the differences among the means are statistically significant, with df (4,75) and p = .001. A similar result was found with Form A.

Relation to Medical Diagnosis

An analysis was made of the scores of the subjects in terms of the medical diagnosis of mild, moderate and severe involvement. The means in succession were 17.9 ± 5.7, 19.3 ± 5.1 and 19.0 ± 5.2. An analysis of variance indicated that the differences among the means are slight. F = 1.16, df (2,220), and p = 30%. This result also is consistent with that of Form A.

There remains the task of evaluating the relations of sound discrimination scores to several other variables. These concern the relation of test scores to chronological age, mental age and IQ, the effect of the position of sounds in words, the effect of spasticity and athetosis, and the effect of the extent of paralysis.

Relation of Test Scores to Chronological Age, Mental Age and IQ

While the correlation value for chronological age and mental age are significant at the 1% level, the coefficients of forecasting efficiency are only 5% and 14%. The correlation of .42 with IQ is not significant.

Effect of Position in Words

The means and standard deviations of the sounds in the initial, medial and final positions in the words were calculated in order to learn if position is a significant factor. Using a table of random numbers, five items were drawn from the list of pairs in Table 61 to equalize the number of items in the three positions. The mean for initials was 4.1, for medials 3.3 and for finals 4.2. The standard deviations all were 1.2.

In the corresponding problem in Form A, it was reported that the mean for the initial position was greater than that of the final position. In order to resolve the confusion Form A was replicated on a sample of 260 children. The means of the initial and final positions on this group turned out to be alike. Thus it is evident that as far as positions of the sounds in the pairs of words are concerned the findings resulting from Form A and B are similar. This, it should be emphasized, contrasts with the findings in regard to articulation where initials exceed finals in mean value.

Effect of Spasticity and Athetosis

The means of spastics, athetoids and mixed cases are 19.8 ± 4.4 for the first, 19.6 ± 4.4 for the second and 18.4 ± 4.3 for the mixed category. As with Form A, the difference between the means of spastics and athetoids on Form B is not significant.

Effect of Extent of Paralysis

The extent of paralysis is indicated by similar means. Quadriplegics make a mean of 19.5 ± 4.9 on Form B and paraplegics a score of 20.4 ± 4.7. It is obvious that there is very little difference between these values. This result is consistent with that found with Form A.

The means for right and left hemiplegia again are alike. For the right hemiplegics it is 18.7 ± 4.7, and for the left it is 19.0 ± 5.6. The same result was found with other types of data.

Summary

This is a project on the construction and standardization of a parallel sound discrimination test (Form B). It is designed for use with cerebral palsied children from age 6 through 16 years. The reliability of the test using a Kuder-Richardson formula is r = .88. Further evidence of the internal consistency of the data is that the means of two widely different geographical samples are the same, the variances are homogeneous and differences between boys and girls are not significant. Using the method of extreme groups for evaluating the validity of Form B, the difference between the means of the scores of extreme chronological age groups was found to be statistically significant. The difference between the means of sound discrimination scores of children rated very good and very poor in general language ability was also significant. The correlation of chronologic age and sound discrimination scores was r = .32, of mental age and scores r = .43, and the correlation of IQ and scores was .11. There was a significant chronological age progression in the scores; there was a significant mental age progression in the scores; the effect of position of sounds in words is inconclusive. The means of scores of children diagnosed medically as mild, moderate and severe were alike. The extent of physical paralysis had no effect on the means of the sound discriminations of quadriplegics, hemiplegics and paraplegics. The means of right and left hemiplegics are alike.

Chapter 36

A Comparison of Sound Discrimination of Mentally Retarded and Cerebral Palsied Children

T HE PURPOSE OF this investigation is to study the sound discrimination ability of mentally retarded children and to compare it with that of cerebral palsied children. The report is divided into two parts. The first concerns the reliability and validity of Form A* using mentally retarded children as subjects. The second part presents some results obtained with the test. The specific aims of the study are to determine the reliability of a sound discrimination test (Form A), when used with mentally retarded children; to determine the validity of Form A when used with mentally retarded cases; to learn if there are sex differences; to determine the effect of chronological age; to compare the ability of educables and trainables to discriminate sounds; to determine the relation of sound discrimination scores to vocabulary scores; to compare the difficulties of the items of Form A for mentally retarded and cerebral palsied children; to determine the differences in sound discrimination ability among the types of mental retardation; and to compare the mean scores of mentally retarded and cerebral palsied children.

Sex Differences

Using Form A the means and standard deviation of sound discrimination scores of mentally retarded boys and girls were determined. The mean of 110 boys was found to be 15.3 ± 5.9. For fifty-six girls it was 14.3 ± 6.6. The difference is 1.00, $t = .75$ and $p = .45$. The difference between the means of the sexes is not significant. The two groups therefore belong to the same population of scores and in subsequent analyses the scores may be combined.

---

*With the collaboration of Don D. Hammill.

RESULTS
Part I

Reliability of Sound Discrimination Test Form A

A Kuder-Richardson coefficient of reliability of Form A when administered to 166 mentally retarded children was .87. This value is comparable to the reliability coefficient found with cerebral palsied children, which was also .87.

Validity of Form A in Terms of Three Criteria

The validity of a test is determined in terms of an external criterion. This may be another sound discrimination test or it may be done by the method of extreme groups.

Relation to the Templin Test

First the sound discrimination scores will be compared with those derived from another test. The Templin Sound Discrimination Test (1957) and Form A were both administered to fifty-two mentally retarded children. The Templin test was modified in two ways. Items in it which are duplicates of items in Form A were eliminated. Items in the Templin test in which vowels are paired instead of consonants also were dropped to bring it in line with Form A which is a consonant test. In this manner the Templin test was reduced to fifty items. The coefficient of correlation between the two tests was $r = .83$. This value is significant at the 1% level and may be considered to be evidence for the validity of Form A. Analyses using the method of extreme groups will provide further evidence of the validity of the test.

Relation to Chronological Age

The effect of chronological age on the sound discrimination scores of mentally retarded children is revealed in a progression of scores from 10.1 ± 4.1 for the 9 to 10 year level to 16.3 ± 7.3 for the 15 to 16 year level. It is apparent that there is a chronological age trend in the scores. The older the mentally retarded children the better sound discrimination becomes. In order to learn if the trend is significant, an analysis of variance was done. The probability value was .001.

Relation to Educational Status

The next table gives the comparative data of mentally retarded children who have been rated educable and trainable. Educables are defined as those with IQs above 50 and trainables as those below 50.

The difference between the means of the educables and trainables is significant. The variances are homogeneous.

The evidence for validity from the correlation of the scores of Form A with those of the Templin Sound Discrimination Test, together with the evidence yielded by the method of extreme groups—namely, chronological age and educational status—seem to be quite adequate. This result is comparable to a similar finding with Form A when used with cerebral palsied children. Inasmuch as the reliability and validity of Form A, which was originally standardized for use with cerebral palsied children, are both adequate, this form may be used also to test the sound discrimination ability of mentally retarded children.

Part II

Part II will report a number of results from the administration of Form A. They include the relation of sound discrimination scores to vocabulary, to chronological age and to IQ, a comparison of difficulties of sound discrimination scores of mentally retarded and cerebral palsied children, the means scores of mental retardation, and a comparison of the means of scores of mentally retarded and cerebral palsied children.

Relation to Vocabulary

The Peabody Picture Vocabulary Test and Form A were administered to fifty-two mentally retarded children. The Pearson r was .26. Since the coefficient of determination (r^2) amounts to only 7%, the effect of vocabulary ability of the children on their sound discrimination quite apparently is not very strong.

TABLE 64

Means and Standard Deviations of Sound Discrimination Test (Form A) of Educable and Trainable Mentally Retarded Children

	N	M	σ	diff	t	df	p
Educables	119	15.6	6.5				
Trainables	37	11.5	5.6	4.1	3.25	154	.001

Relation to Chronological Age and IQ

The correlations of chronological age and IQ to sound discrimination are r = .26 and .38 and r² = .07 and .14. These are weak relationships.

In order to compare these results with those obtained with cerebral palsied children, the following values are presented. The *r* for chronological age is .52, a moderate correlation. The *r* for IQ is .33. The *r²'s* amount to .27 and .11. These are not substantial values. This means that the ability to discriminate sounds by mentally retarded and cerebral palsied children can hardly be predicted accurately from chronological age or from IQ.

TABLE 65

Orders of Difficulty of Items of Sound Discrimination Test (Form A) for Mentally Retarded and Cerebral Palsied Children

		% of Passes	
	Item	*MR (N=167)*	*CP (N=260)*
1.	tin-*th*in	75	84
2.	*l*ate-*d*ate	75	87
3.	*p*ig-*b*ig	74	83
5.	test-tex*t*	63	80
6.	bu*d*-bu*g*	57	68
7.	*ch*ip-*sh*ip	54	72
8.	habita*t*-habita*nt*	60	37
9.	*s*op-*sh*op	65	80
10.	co*n*ical-co*m*ical	40	56
12.	bea*t*s-bea*ds*	60	80
13.	cy*t*ology-psy*ch*ology	38	58
14.	class-clas*p*	49	76
15.	mu*sh*-mu*ch*	63	83
16.	*p*atriarch-*m*atriarch	65	83
18.	*w*ear-*wh*ere	38	40
19.	*b*iscuit-*b*risket	60	79
20.	*f*oal-*st*ole	72	91
21.	pass-pa*th*	49	62
22.	convergent-conver*s*ant	51	81
23.	falls-fal*se*	62	85
25.	re*f*racted-re*tr*acted	66	89
26.	co*k*e-co*p*e	54	82
27.	*c*arrion-*M*arion	74	91
29.	*f*risking-*wh*isking	68	87
30.	*th*igh-*s*igh	65	84

Comparison of Item Difficulties

Table 65 gives the order of difficulty for mentally retarded and cerebral palsied children.

By inspection it will be noted at once that the order of difficulty of the items for the two groups of children is different. The principle in reading the table is that the smaller the percent of passes, the more difficult the item is. For instance the most difficult pair of sounds for the mentally retarded is number 13, "cytology-psychology," the percent is 38. The corresponding percent for this pair for cerebral palsied children is 58. For the cerebral palsied children the most difficult item is number 8, "habitat-habitant," with a percentage of 37. For mentally retarded children, it is 60%. Again item number 26, "coke-cope," is easy for the cerebral palsied children but only moderately so the mentally retarded children. The "tin-thin," was passed by only 75% of the mentally retarded children in contrast to 84% by cerebral palsied children. On the whole the orders of difficulty are quite dissimilar as indicated in this table. This points up the principle that there is no single order of difficulty of sound discrimination items, but that it varies with the type of child and his handicap.

Table 66 gives the mean percent of all items passed by the two groups. The table shows that on the average more cerebral palsied children pass the items of the test than mentally retarded children. This means that the cerebral palsied children are somewhat more successful with sound discrimination than mentally retarded children. On the other hand, with articulation, it was earlier found mentally retarded children exceeded cerebral palsied children.

SUMMARY

One hundred and sixty-six mentally retarded children from 6

TABLE 66
Percent of Sound Discrimination Items of Form A Passed by Mentally Retarded and Cerebral Palsied Children

	N	M	Range
Mentally Retarded	166	60	38–75
Cerebral Palsied	260	76	37–91

to 17 years of age were examined with a Form A of a Sound Discrimination Test originally designed for use with cerebral palsied children. The subjects were from the states of Arkansas, California, Colorado, Connecticut, Kansas, Missouri and West Virginia. It was found that there were no significant differences between the means of the sexes. When a Kuder-Richardson coefficient of reliability was applied to the data the r was .87. The validity of the test was determined by correlating it with the Templin Sound Discrimination Test. The coefficient of correlation between the two tests was .83. The inference is that Form A is suitable for use with mentally retarded children. There was a significant trend in the scores with chronological age. Educational status is a factor. Educables made a significantly higher mean score than trainables. The correlations of chronological age and IQ are low, indicating the small relationship. The order of difficulty of the items of the Sound Discrimination Test are not the same for the mentally retarded and the cerebral palsied. The items of the tests are more difficult for mentally retarded children than for cerebral palsied children. The mean of sound discrimination scores of non–brain-injured mentally retarded children is significantly greater than that of brain-injured children. The mean of the sound discrimination scores of the mentally retarded children on Form A of the test is significantly lower than that of cerebral palsied children.

An Item Analysis of a Sound Discrimination Test of Mentally Retarded Children

IN SEVERAL STUDIES with cerebral palsied children, parallel Forms A and B of a sound discrimination test were administered to groups of these children. The tests were also given to mentally retarded children. However, an item analysis of Form A with the mentally retarded children was not completed. One purpose of the present study was to make such an analysis in terms of discriminating power of the items, their uniqueness and their difficulty. Another purpose was to provide further verification of the reliability and validity of Form A when used with retarded children. A further aim was to investigate the status of a sample of children in Hawaii. The problem of the present investigation, then, is to determine if this test, designed for use with cerebral palsied children, is suitable for use with mentally retarded children. When Form A was used with cerebral palsied cases the reliability coefficient was .87. Observer reliability was 96%.

PROCEDURE

The subjects of the present investigation were seventy-six mentally retarded children from the state of Hawaii and from states in the northwest mainland. The mean chronological age was 12 years, 5 months, and the range was 6 to 17 years. The adequacy of hearing of the children was determined by an audiometer or by a spondee test. The criterion was ability to hear in a conversational setting. The diagnoses of mental retardation were taken from medical records at the various facilities. The following medical classification was based on these records.

	F	%
Nonbrain Injured	34	45
Brain Injured	25	33
Hydrocephalic	1	1
Epileptic	3	4
Undetermined	13	17
	76	100

The first problem was to determine if the scores of the boys and girls in the two regions could be pooled. If there were no significant differences among them then the scores could be treated as a whole. The means and standard deviations are presented in Table 67.

Results of an analysis of variance indicated that differences between the Hawaiian and Northwest states and between sexes were not significant. In other words, mentally retarded children in Hawaii are on a par with those on the mainland in sound discrimination. Accordingly the data were pooled in order to perform subsequent analyses.

Item Analysis

The item analysis was made in terms of the three criteria of discriminating power, of uniqueness and of difficulty. It is presented in Table 68.

On the whole the items meet the three criteria of the item analysis. However, it is seen that seven of the twenty-five coefficients of discriminating power are less than .50. For instance, item 8 has a low discriminating power, but the values for uniqueness and difficulty are satisfactory. It has thus a degree of usefulness as a test item. Similar evaluations may be made of items 21 and 22. In spite of these limitations the mean coefficient of discriminating power is well above .50. The phi coefficients for uniqueness are all low with a mean of .22, and the percents of difficulty range from 33 to 86 with a mean of 64%.

TABLE 67

Means and Standard Deviations of Scores on Form A of a Sound Discrimination Test of Mentally Retarded Children According to Sex and Regions

Regions	Boys			Girls		
	N	M	σ	N	M	σ
Northwest	12	16.3	5.9	8	15.4	6.5
Hawaii	26	16.0	4.6	30	16.2	5.2

TABLE 68

**Item Analysis of Sound Discrimination Test (Form A) of
Mentally Retarded Children**

Item*	Discriminating Power r	Mean Uniqueness φ	Difficulty %
1	40	7	74
2	62	12	84
3	75	16	76
5	53	11	63
6	78	20	63
7	57	12	46
8	20	6	50
9	82	25	63
10	60	26	53
12	72	28	66
13	60	23	39
14	70	25	57
15	81	25	71
16	74	26	78
18	44	3	34
19	70	33	71
20	41	9	86
21	36	20	33
22	25	34	68
23	44	17	63
24	79	42	72
26	59	26	72
27	74	28	78
29	64	50	78
30	70		67
	M = .60	M = .22	M = 64%
	Range = .20–.81	Range = .03–.50	Range = 33–86%

* The items corresponding to the numbers are found in Chart 17.

Reliability of the Test

The reliability of this test was determined also by means of the Kuder-Richardson formula No. 20. The coefficient of reliability of Form A of the test using mentally retarded subjects is .81. This value is comparable to the reliability coefficient found with cerebral palsied children where r was .87. Concerning parallel form reliability the means of Form A and B using mentally retarded children were 18.3 and 18.2. The standard deviations were 5.4 and 5.2. The correlation was $r = 80$. Thus the two forms yield equivalent results.

Validity of the Test

The method of extreme groups was used to evaluate the validity of the sound discrimination test when used with mentally retarded children. Variables on which the extreme groups were selected are (1) vocabulary, (2) abstraction and (3) mental classification.

The method of extreme groups was applied to the upper and lower scores of the Peabody Picture Vocabulary Test (PPVT), which was administered to the children. These groups each included 27% of the scores, a principle used by Flanagan (1939) for the selection of test items. Here it is arbitrarily used to select members of the extreme groups. The upper mean is 18.8, the lower is 14.2. Variances are homogeneous. The difference between the means of these extreme groups was significant at the .001 level.

Another variable on the basis on which two extreme groups were selected is the ability of the children to perform the mental process of abstraction. The mean of sound discrimination scores of children who ranked high on an abstraction test was compared with the mean of children who ranked low on it. The mean of the upper 27% of the cases is 19.8 ± 3.0. For the lower it is 12.5 ± 4.4. The difference between these means is also significant at the .001 level.

IQs of the subjects were secured from records at various facilities. The mental tests most frequently used by the local psychologists were the Wechsler Intelligence Scale for Children (WISC) and the Revised Stanford-Binet. The following classification of mental retardation was made according to the American Association on Mental Deficiency (Heber, 1961). Seventy-one IQ scores were available.

Classification	IQ	F	%
Borderline	70–84	24	34
Mild Retardation	55–69	31	44
Moderate Retardation	40–54	15	21
Severe Retardation	25–39	1	1
		71	100

An analysis of variance was done on three classifications—borderline, mild and moderate retardation. One severely re-

TABLE 69

**Means and Standard Deviations of Sound Discrimination Scores (Form A)
of Mentally Retarded Children by Mental Age Levels According to the
Classification of AAMD**

Classification	N	M	σ
Borderline	24	19.2	4.4
Mild	31	15.6	5.0
Moderate	16	12.8	4.5

tarded case was included in the moderate group. The values were
presented in Table 69.

Since the F ratio was significant at the .001 level, the means of
the extreme groups, the borderline and the moderate, differ significantly, affording further evidence of the validity of Form A.

RESULTS

There were no significant sex differences in the scores of the
mentally retarded children. There were no significant differences
between the performance of mentally retarded children in the
state of Hawaii and children in the states on the mainland. The
mean discrimination power was $r = .60$. A majority of these values
exceeded $r = .50$. Some however were low. The mean phi coefficient of uniqueness was $\phi = .22$, the range was $\phi = .03$ to .50.
The mean percent of difficulty was 64, the range was from 33%
to 86%. The Kuder-Richardson coefficient of test reliability was
.81. The percent of interobserver reliability was 98%. Validity,
using the method of extreme groups based on three criteria, was
adequate.

CONCLUSION

The purpose of this study was to complete an item analysis of
a sound discrimination test, Form A. Evidence was provided that
in general Form A, in this respect, is adequate for use with mentally retarded children. In addition, an aim was to provide verification of the reliability and validity of Form A. In a previous
investigation it had been found that the reliability and validity
were adequate when used with mentally retarded children. The
present study confirms this finding. The scores of mentally retarded children in Hawaii are not exceptional. This concludes
the development of the construct of sound discrimination. The
next construct to be considered is that of abstraction.

PART III
ABSTRACTION

The process of abstracting and categorizing meanings or referents are characteristic higher mental activities. The normal human being depends on and performs them continuously during his working hours. They are based on the ability to discriminate and are among the most ubiquitous of the cognitive processes. Not only are they an ubiquitous process, but they are tremendously important in daily living. For if we were required to respond to each event in our lives as unique, we would have to learn each time what to do about it. Soon the bewildering array of environmental events would overwhelm us. It is, therefore, important to know to what extent the speech handicapped child is disadvantaged in respect to this communication variable.

Chapter 38

An Abstraction Test

~~~~~~

THE PURPOSE OF this study is to construct and standardize a parallel form test which may be used to evaluate the ability of these children to perform the processes of abstraction.

ABSTRACTING AND CATEGORIZING

First something should be said by way of definition. Abstraction and categorization are related or complimentary mental activities. Abstraction implies categorization of some kind. The term "abstraction" generally may be defined as a response to a property or an attribute isolated from its context or from a group. The group or the category may take several forms. The categories of things, events or attributes which are used in the present study may be described as sequential, coordinate and mixed.

A sequential category or context may be illustrated in the arrangement of playing cards. Three cards numbered 5, 6 and 7 of hearts illustrate a sequential category. It is recognized or categorized by card players as a book. A variation of the sequential category may occur in response to the question, "What number among the following is less than six: 9, 8, 5, 10?" Here the term "less than" is the abstract term. In this instance the subject performs the process of selecting one from a context of unlike terms.

The coordinate category includes terms which are similar in rank. Thus in a deck of cards, four kings constitute such a category. The members of a coordinate category have a common property not found outside the category. For instance in the context cat, dog, horse, tree, three members form a category called animal while tree is outside the category.

A third type, for want of a better term, may be called the

Note: This study was conducted and written with the collaboration of Don D. Hammill.

mixed category. It refers to a context which includes unrelated objects or events. It has two forms. In one form, although its members may have no common attribute, one member may be specified by an abstract term outside the context. This form may be illustrated by the following. "Which is hardest: cloth, grass, iron, water?" The abstract quality is hardness which lies outside the context. Another form reverses this situation. Members of the context all may be abstract categories of which a concrete term or object outside the context may be an instance. To illustrate: "A rabbit is: tall, furry, feathery, prickly?" The outside object is a rabbit which belongs to the category of furriness.

The items of the Abstraction Test have been selected to illustrate these forms of categorization and abstraction.

PROCEDURE

A pool of one hundred abstract and categorization items was assembled and divided into two groups of fifty items each. They were designated as preliminary Forms X and Y. Form X was administered to 125 cerebral palsied children ranging in age from 6 to 17 years in nine southern and southeastern states. They were Alabama, Arkansas, Florida, Georgia, Louisiana, Mississippi, Oklahoma, South Carolina and Texas. Preliminary Form Y was administered to another sample of 124 children of the same age range in the same region. An item analysis consisting of the discriminating power of the items, their uniqueness and their difficulty was done on the data.

Table 70 summarizes the analysis of items in preliminary Forms X and Y.

It is interesting to note that the two means in each column are about the same. Also it is seen that the ranges of correlation for the discriminating power are well above the cutting value of r = .50 and that those for uniqueness are below the cutting value.

TABLE 70
Analysis of Items of Preliminary Forms X and Y of the Abstraction Test

| | Discriminating Power | | Uniqueness | | % Difficulty | |
	Mean r	Range	Mean ϕ	Range	Mean	Range
Form X	.80	.63–.90	.34	.22–.39	63	42–83
Form Y	.79	.61–.90	.37	.30–.47	62	40–84

The ranges for percent of difficulty are from 40 to 84. It is permissible then to conclude that the item analyses of the two preliminary forms of the abstraction test in general satisfy the three criteria.

The method of selcting the twenty-five items for each of the final forms was to examine the three criterion values for each item. The items which best met the criteria were selected and incorporated in the final forms. For instance item 1 in Table 71, Form X, had a discriminating power of r = .73 which is greater than the cutting r of .50. It had a uniqueness value of r = .31 which is less than the cutting r of .50. It had a difficulty value of 63%. Since this item meets the three criteria it was in-

TABLE 71
Final Form X
Abstraction Test for Use with Cerebral Palsied Children

Item*	Discriminating Power r	Uniqueness φ	Difficulty %
1	73	31	63
2	87	35	75
3	73	30	43
4	82	37	69
5	77	39	60
6	84	39	66
7	90	36	76
8	81	32	54
9	77	32	54
10	77	38	74
11	77	27	46
12	88	31	64
13	83	38	57
14	87	36	59
15	86	30	67
16	82	33	83
17	74	37	70
18	85	33	66
19	82	31	70
20	72	33	65
21	84	22	42
22	82	27	47
23	63	38	57
24	71	43	66
25	84	39	69

* The items of Form X to which the numbers correspond are found in Chart 22.

TABLE 72
Final Form Y
Abstraction Test for Use with Cerebral Palsied Children

Item*	Discriminating Power r	Uniqueness φ	Difficulty %
1	73	36	63
2	78	37	54
3	82	39	66
4	84	40	46
5	90	44	46
6	84	38	59
7	81	38	68
8	86	42	90
9	88	40	62
10	83	34	40
11	87	38	50
12	86	39	62
13	71	35	75
14	74	35	75
15	85	39	72
16	74	36	79
17	72	30	84
18	84	34	68
19	71	32	65
20	61	30	43
21	82	47	64
22	63	39	51
23	69	41	65
24	71	36	44
25	84	36	64

* The items of Form Y to which the numbers correspond are found in Chart 23.

cluded in the final Form X of the test.

Table 71 includes the items selected for Final Form X on the basis of the three criteria.

Table 72 includes the items selected for Final Form Y.

Instruction to the Examiner

The final form of test X together with instructions for the administration are found in Chart 14 in the Appendix. The instructions are given verbally. In no case is any deviation from the specified instructions permitted without jeopardizing the validity of the test results.

While the examiner must adhere to the strictest conformity in administering the test, the subject may respond in any manner

possible to him (verbally, manually, or both). Most cerebral palsied children are able to respond verbally; however, occasionally
allowances in the response pattern must be made for children
whose physical involvements are such that a verbal response is not
possible.

From time to time, a child will be too physically involved even
for the moderate motor control required to successfully accomplish the technique just mentioned. These children can respond
with eye blinks or gross muscular movements. One method found
useful is for the examiner to hold the child's arm gently and request him to move the arm as his response to the correct choice.

The use of these techniques enables the examiner to test many
children who would otherwise be labeled "untestable." These
procedures also allow the mental function called abstracting ability to be measured without the confusing influence of the
associated physical disability.

RESULTS

The two final forms of the test were administered to two more
samples of cerebral palsied children. One sample was from a num-
ber of northeastern states, the other from the southwestern states.
The states included in the two samples are Arizona, California,
Colorado, Connecticut, Maine, Massachusetts, New Hampshire,
New Mexico, New York, Pennsylvania, Utah and Vermont.

Reliability of the Observer

Two observers recorded independently the responses of fifty-
five children with speech problems; both forms of the Abstraction
Test were administered. Seventeen cerebral palsied children received Form X and fifteen Form Y. Seven articulatory cases were
given Form X and five Form Y. The tests were administered to a
number of other children diagnosed as mentally retarded and
aphasic. In addition there was a cleft palate case and a stutterer.

The overall percent of agreement on the fifty-five children
amounted to 98.6. This means that there is about a 2% error in
the data.

Administration of the Final Forms

Previous to the administration of the test the children's hearing was evaluated by an audiometric test. A sweep at 15 db of frequencies of 500, 1000, 2000 and 4000 was used. Also a short list of spondees and directions were used as a further check on the adequacy of hearing. With children who had been given an audiometric by the local audiologist, only the list of spondaic words and directions was used. Accordingly the factor of the hearing of the subjects was controlled. Children with hearing losses were not used in the experiment.

Form X of the Abstraction Test was next administered to the subject. It was followed by the Peabody Picture Vocabulary Test and then by Form Y. The second subject was first given Form Y, then the Similarities Test from the WISC followed by Form X. The order of administration of the two forms was then alternated from subject to subject. In this manner, the factor of fatigue was equalized. With this procedure all the children took both forms of the Abstraction Test, but half of them were given the Peabody between the two forms and the other half the Similarities Test from the WISC.

Sex and Geographical Differences

In order to learn if there are geographical and sex differences, an analysis of variance was done. The means and standard deviations are given in Table 73 for Form X.

Interaction was not present in a two-way analysis of variance. The differences between the means of sexes as well as between regions were not significant.

The means and standard deviations of scores on Form Y are presented in Table 74.

The analysis of variance of the scores on test Form Y also indicated that the difference between the means of the sexes are not significant. The same holds also for differences between the means of the regions. Since the differences among the means are not

TABLE 73
Means and Standard Deviations of Abstraction Test (Form X)
Scores of Boys and Girls in Two Geographical Areas

	Boys			Girls		
	N	M	σ	N	M	σ
Northeast	49	16.1	8.4	42	17.5	8.7
Southwest	29	17.4	6.9	22	14.6	6.7

TABLE 74
**Means and Standard Deviations of Abstraction Test (Form Y)
Scores of Boys and Girls in Two Geographical Areas**

	Boys			Girls		
	N	M	σ	N	M	σ
Northeast	49	16.7	8.0	42	17.8	8.6
Southwest	29	17.6	7.8	22	16.1	7.0

significant the four groups may be considered to belong to the same population.

Reliability of the Abstraction Test

The reliability of the test was determined in two ways, one was parallel form reliability and the other, the method of rational equivalence. Parallel forms of a test should have approximately equal means, their variances should be homogeneous, and the correlation between them should be substantial. The second method used in determining the reliability of the test was to apply a Kuder-Richardson formula to the data.

The mean score of Form X is 16.6, that of Form Y is 17.1. The means of the two forms thus are approximately equal. The variance of the scores of Form X is 59.5, that of Form Y is 60.0. The variances are seen to be homogeneous. The correlation between the scores of the 142 children on the two forms is .95. The Abstraction Test thus meets adequately the three criteria for test equivalence; consequently it would make no difference which form of the test would be used for retesting purposes.

When the Kuder-Richardson formula No. 20 was applied to the data of Form X the coefficient of reliability was .95. For Form Y the coefficient was .96. It may be pointed out that the reliability of each form is further attested by the closeness of their mean scores in the two preceding tables.

Validity of the Abstraction Test

The concept of validity is concerned with the correlation of a test with other information about the subjects taking the test. The concept of validity thus is based on an external criterion with the limitation that the external criteria must be other data about the subjects tested.

Types of information against which test scores can be validated are the Wechsler Similarities Test and the Peabody Vocabulary Test. The items of the Similarities Test are concerned with the problem of abstraction. Presumably then it is a suitable instrument with which to validate the present test. Form X correlates $r = .74$ with the WISC Similarities Test, and Form Y correlates with it with an $r = .72$.

The correlations of the two forms with the Abstraction Test are seen to correlate in the lower seventies with the Similarities Test. The probability values are at the 1% level.

The Abstraction Tests correlate with the scores of the Peabody Picture Vocabulary Test with $r = .73$ and $.79$. The correlations are significant at the 1% level. It is apparent that when the forms of the Abstraction Test are correlated with the two external criteria—namely, the Similarities Test and the Peabody Picture Vocabulary Test—the coefficients of correlation are of a size which may be accepted as evidence for the validity of the test.

From the statistical analysis, both the reliability and the validity of the Abstraction Test is acceptable for use with cerebral palsied children between the ages of 6 and 17 years.

SUMMARY

The purpose of this study is to construct and standardize a parallel form test which may be used to evaluate the ability of cerebral palsied children to perform the mental processes of abstraction and categorization. The term "abstraction" generally may be defined as a response to a property or attribute isolated from its context. A pool of abstract items was assembled into two groups designated as preliminary Forms X and Y. Form X was administered to 125 cerebral palsied children between the ages of 6 and 17 years in nine southern and southeastern states. Form Y was administered to a second sample of 124 children in the same region. An item analysis consisting of the discriminating power of the items, their uniqueness and their difficulty was done. The final forms of the test were composed of twenty-five items each selected on the basis of the three criteria. They were then administered to 142 cerebral palsied children in twelve states in the northeast and the southwest parts of the country.

Observer reliability was determined of fifty-five subjects. The percent of agreement amounted to 98. Significant sex differences in abstract ability were not present. Regional differences were not found. Since the differences between the means of the two forms was not significant and since the variances were homogeneous and the correlations between the forms were substantial, the two forms may be considered to be equivalent. When a Kuder-Richardson formula was applied to Form X, the reliability coefficient amounted to .95. For Form Y, it was .96. Validity of the test was determined by correlating the scores on Form X with the WISC Similarities Test. The r was .74. For Form Y, the correlation was .72. The scores of the Abstraction Test were also correlated with the vocabulary scores of the Peabody Picture Vocabulary Test. For Form X, r = .73, and for Form Y, r = .79. It may be concluded that the reliability and validity of the Abstraction Test are adequate for use with cerebral palsied children between the ages of 6 and 17 years.

Chapter 39

Some Results with an Abstraction Test

IN THE PREVIOUS CHAPTER an item analysis and the reliability and validity of an Abstraction Test for use with cerebral palsied children between the ages of 6 and 17 years were reported. The present study is an investigation of the relationship between the ability of these crippled children to perform abstract functions and the extent, degree and type of their paralytic involvement, mental age, chronological age and therapist ratings of general speech and language ability. A description of the subjects and of Form X of the test are found in the Appendix.

RESULTS

Effect of Extent of Paralysis

The mean scores by quadriplegics, hemiplegics and paraplegics on the two forms of the Abstraction Test were found to cluster around 7.0 ± 3.9. An analysis of variance indicated that significant differences do not exist either among the three groups or between the two forms.

Effect of Degree of Physical Disability

The mean scores on the two forms of mildly, moderately and severely involved cerebral palsied children were found to be 15.6 ± 7.4, 17.4 ± 8.1 and 16.7 ± 8.5. An analysis of variance was performed on the data. The differences among the means were not significant. Thus the degree of physical disability is not a factor affecting the ability of these children to perform the process of abstraction. Since Form Y correlates with Form X, a comparable analysis of variance was not performed on its data.

Note: This study was conducted and written with the collaboration of Don D. Hammill.

Effect of Type of Paralysis

A comparison of the mean scores of spastics and athetoids was made. The mean for ninety spastics was 16.4 ± 8.0 and for athetoids it was 18.3 ± 7.2. The difference between the means of spastics and athetoids on Form X of the Abstraction Test is not significant. Since there is no significant difference between the means of spastics and athetoids, nor among the means of quadriplegics, hemiplegics and paraplegics, nor among those rated mild, moderate and severe, the inference may be drawn that physical disability is not a deterrent to the use of this test with this type of child.

Relation to Mental Age

The mental ages of the seventy-one children were determined by means of the Peabody Picture Vocabulary Test. The correlations are $r = .70$ for Form X and $.76$ for Form Y. These correlations are significant at the 1% level.

Relation to Chronological Age

The chronological ages and the scores of the Abstraction Test were correlated. The values for two samples were calculated. They are $r = .30$ with Form X and $.26$ with Form Y. Although they are significant at the $.01$ level, the coefficients of forecasting efficiency indicate that the predictive efficiencies of these r's range from 3% to 5%. This means that chronological age is not a very dependable basis for judging the abstract ability of the cerebral palsied child.

Relation to Therapists' Ratings

A trend is apparent in the scores of very good, good, medium, poor and very poor. It progressed from 13.4 ± 9.6 for very poor to 20.8 ± 4.6. An analysis of variance yielded an F ratio of 2.75, df $(4,137)$ and $p = .025$. The significant trend in the mean scores of the data therefore may be taken as evidence for the validity of the test.

SUMMARY

In this study an Abstraction Test was used to investigate the ability of 142 cerebral palsied children to perform abstract functions in their relation to the extent, the degree and type of paralytic involvement and their relation to mental age, chronological age and therapists' ratings of general speech and language ability. The test yielded the following results.

The differences among the means of quadriplegics, hemiplegics and paraplegics in abstract ability were not significant. The differences among the means of mildly, moderately and severely involved cerebral palsied children were not significant. The correlation of abstract scores and mental age scores on Form X of the test is .70 and Form Y it is .76. The correlation of chronological age and the scores on Forms X and Y for two samples of the children ranged from $r = .24$ to $r = .30$. The correlations of general speech and language ability and the ability of the cerebral palsied children are .28 and .29.

It seems reasonable to infer from these findings that (1) physical disability as such is not a deterrent to use of the Abstraction Test with cerebral palsied children, (2) chronological age is not a dependable factor for judging the abstract ability of this type of child, (3) therapists' ratings of the status of the speech and language ability is not a good predictor of the children's abstract ability and (4) among the several variables in this study the mental ability of these children is the only important factor in the process.

Chapter 40

An Abstraction Test Adapted for Use with Mentally Retarded Children

THE PROCESSES OF abstracting and categorizing attributes, objects and events are characteristically higher mental activities. They underlie many communication episodes. They are of great importance in daily adjustments and are among the most ubiquitous of the cognitive processes. Therefore it is of considerable interest to learn to what degree the mentally retarded child is handicapped in respect to the processes of abstraction.

The present study is a sequel to the report in which the construction of an abstraction test for use with cerebral palsied children was described. The problem of this investigation is to determine if the test designed to be used with cerebral palsied children is suitable for use with mentally retarded children. The method of approach was to administer the Abstraction Test to a group of mentally retarded children and to perform a series of operations on the data. The operations again are concerned with (1) an item analysis which determines the relative difficulty of the items as well as their discriminating power and their uniqueness, (2) the reliability of the test and (3) the validity of the test.

PROCEDURE

A preliminary pool of items had been administered to cerebral palsied children and subjected to an item analysis. On the basis of this analysis, twenty-five of the items which best met the three criteria were selected for the final form of the test. This form was used in the present project. The rationale of the procedure is that if the item analysis criteria are satisfactorily met by the data secured from mentally retarded children and if the reliability and validity of the test likewise are adequate, then it may be used with confidence to measure the abstracting ability of those children.

RESULTS

Sex and Geographical Differences

An initial analysis was made to determine if the scores of boys and girls in the two regions could be pooled. The result of the analysis indicated that the differences either between regions or between sexes were not significant. Since no evidence was found for sex and geographical differences, the data may be pooled in subsequent analyses.

TABLE 75
Item Analysis Abstraction Test (Form X) for Mentally Retarded Children

Item*	Discriminating Power r	Mean Uniqueness φ	Difficulty %
1	.81	.34	44
2	.96	.40	67
3	.88	.33	46
4	.96	.28	67
5	.96	.35	53
6	.92	.24	74
7	1.00	.17	84
8	.81	.24	59
9	.96	.37	39
10	.99	.33	70
11	.85	.30	46
12	.92	.26	59
13	.96	.37	56
14	.88	.26	55
15	.96	.33	71
16	1.00	.23	88
17	.96	.32	75
18	1.00	.29	72
19	1.00	.29	73
20	.88	.29	56
21	.58	.32	22
22	.85	.38	37
23	.62	.38	41
24	1.00	.40	52
25	.88	—	58
	Mean = .90	Mean = .31	Mean = 59
	Range: .58–1.00	Range: .17–.40	Range: 22–88

* The items corresponding to the numbers are found in Chart 22.

Item Analysis

The purpose of this particular analysis is to determine if the items of Form X of the Abstraction Test are suitable for use with mentally retarded children. The values resulting from the item analysis are presented in Table 75. It includes discriminating power, uniqueness and percent of difficulty. The mean for discriminating power is .90, for uniqueness the mean of the means is .31. Thus the criterion that discriminating power value should be higher than those of uniqueness has been met in these data.

The values presented in Table 76 permit comparisons to be made between the results of the item analyses obtained for mentally retarded and cerebral palsied subjects.

It is seen that the three criteria based on the scores of mentally retarded children are comparable to those of the cerebral palsied children. The discriminating powers exceed the cutting point of r = .50, the uniqueness values are less than r = .50 and percents of difficulty are within the range of 22 and 88. The three criteria based on the scores of mentally retarded children are comparable to those of the cerebral palsied children.

Reliability of the Test

The Kuder-Richardson formula No. 20 was used to assess the reliability of Form X of the test when used with mentally retarded children. The coefficient of reliability was .90. This compares favorably with the coefficient of reliability based on scores of cerebral palsied cases which was .95.

Validity of the Test

The validity of the test was evaluated by means of the method of extreme groups. Three criteria were used. They are (1) chron-

TABLE 76

A Comparison of the Means and Ranges of an Item Analysis of an Abstration Test as Determined on Mentally Retarded and Cerebral Palsied Children

	Discriminating Power r		Mean Uniqueness		Difficulty %	
	M	Range	M	Range	M	Range
Mentally Retarded	.90	.58–1.00	.31	.17–.40	59	22–88
Cerebral Palsied	.80	.71– .90	.34	.22–.43	63	42–83

ological age, (2) the mental classification of the American Association of Mental Deficiency (AAMD) and (3) vocabulary ability.

The Effect of Chronological Age

The trend with chronological age increases from a mean of 10.2 ± 5.1 at the 6 to 9 year level to 16.3 ± 7.4 at the 16 to 17 age level. The trend is significant at p = .01 and provides grounds for the valid use of this test with mentally retarded children.

Relation to IQ

IQs of the subjects were taken from the records at various institutions. The mental tests most frequently used were the WISC and the Revised Stanford-Binet. The following tabulation was made according to AAMD classifications.

The method of extreme groups again was applied to secure further evidence for the validity of the test. In the upper part of Table 77 the extreme groups consist of IQ scores of borderline cases and moderate mental retardates. As the *t* reported in Table 77 is significant at the .001 level, the validity of the measure is supported. The means in the lower part of the table are based on PPTV scores, where *p* also is .001.

Comparison of Mentally Retarded and Cerebral Palsied Children

Two comparisons of the means of abstraction scores by 158 mentally retarded children and 142 cerebral palsied children were made. In one, mental age was broken down into four levels and the means of each level were determined and significance tests were applied. In the second comparison chronological age was divided into four levels and a similar procedure was followed.

TABLE 77

Means and Standard Deviations of Abstract Test (Form X) Scores of Mentally Retarded Children by Mental Age Levels According to the Classification of the AAMD

Classification	M	σ	diff	t	df	p
Borderline	17.1	6.3	—	—	—	—
Moderate	8.8	6.1	8.3	4.80	52	.001
Scores Based on the PPVT						
Upper 27%	21.4	5.2	—	—	—	—
Lower 27%	11.4	4.6	10.0	8.13	50	.001

When the scores were based on the four mental age levels the differences between the means of mentally retarded and cerebral palsied children were found to be nonsignificant. The two groups in terms of mental age are alike.

A somewhat different result was found when the scores were based on chronological age levels. This is shown in the following table.

It is apparent from the table that differences in the ability to classify and abstract concepts do not appear until about the tenth year and then the cerebral palsied children become superior to mentally retarded children.

SUMMARY

The purpose of this study was to determine if an abstraction test constructed for use with cerebral palsied children could be used with mentally retarded children also. The procedure was to make an analysis of the items of Form X in terms of discriminating power, uniqueness and difficulty. It was found that the item analysis values based on the scores of mentally retarded children were comparable to those based on scores of cerebral palsied children. The coefficient of reliability of the test itself was .90. For the cerebral palsied children it was .95. Observer reliability was r = .98. The validity of the test was determined by the method of extreme groups and was found to be satisfactory. It may be concluded that Form X of the Abstraction Test is adequate for use with mentally retarded children between the ages of 6 and 17 years.

It is hardly necessary again to emphasize that the content and processes found in the preceding chapters illuminate an operational construct of abstraction.

TABLE 78

Means and Standard Deviations of Abstraction Scores of Mentally Retarded and Cerebral Palsied Children Based on Chronological Age

| CA | Mentally Retarded | | Cerebral Palsied | | diff | Signif. |
	M	σ	M	σ		
6–7	8.9	7.3	9.1	6.5	0.2	No
8–9	11.8	8.6	13.9	7.5	2.1	No
10–11	14.1	7.1	17.1	3.9	3.0	.05
12–16	14.5	6.9	18.2	5.6	3.7	.001

PART IV
VOCABULARY

Previously it was explained that the meaning of a word is determined by the phoneme, that sound substitutions, omissions and distortions decidedly alter the meaning of a word. A further consideration regarding word mastery by speech handicapped children concerns two types of vocabulary. These are the vocabulary of use or expression and the vocabulary of understanding or comprehension. These two vocabulary types broadly exemplify two criteria of communication. The vocabulary of expression relates to the stimulus side of communication, the vocabulary of comprehension to the discriminating or response aspect of communication.

Chapter 41

Word Equipment of Spastic and Athetoid Children

IN EARLIER CHAPTERS, the phonetic equipment of spastic, athetoid and tension athetoid children was analyzed. It was found that significant differences were not present. The present chapter is concerned with the presence of words in the speech of spastic, athetoid and tension athetoid children from 1 to 12 years of age, with the purpose of discovering if there are significant differences in word mastery among the three groups.

PROCEDURE

The data were collected live on the spontaneous speech of 266 subjects in Iowa, Illinois, South Dakota, Kansas, Texas, New York, Maryland and California. Of the 266 children with cerebral palsy, 128 were spastic, 86 were athetoid and 52 were tension athetoid. The record for each subject consisted of his vocalizations uttered on a sample of thirty breath pulsations. The data analyzed in this report are of two kinds: (1) words correctly pronounced and (2) word approximations.

The reliability of the observer in transcribing words was reported in a study by McCurry and Irwin (1953). Using Festinger's formula (1944), the agreement between two observers was 91%. In the McCurry-Irwin study, the distinction between words correctly spoken and words approximately pronounced was defined as follows: "A standard word is defined in terms of its phonetic listing in Kenyon and Knott's *Pronouncing Dictionary of American English*" (1951); and "A word approximation is defined as a phonetic pattern which is interpreted by the observers at the time of transcription as an attempt by the subject to pronounce a standard word. The word approximation is delimited further as a phonetic pattern in which one or more of the phonetic elements of the standard word, either vowel or consonantal elements, are present. This means that some elements of the standard pat-

TABLE 79
Mean Correct Words of Children with Cerebral Palsy

CA	Spastic		Athetoid		Tension Athetoid	
	N	Mean	N	Mean	N	Mean
1–2	22	1.6	6	3.7	6	2.0
3–4	40	5.9	27	3.1	8	2.3
5–6	26	7.0	25	5.5	14	4.4
7–8	23	6.4	10	4.7	11	5.9
9–10	9	8.4	10	7.5	9	12.6
11–12	8	8.8	8	1.9	4	5.2

tern are omitted, and other elements are substituted or added."
This distinction will be used to analyze the word equipment of
children with cerebral palsy. Accordingly, separate analyses will
be made of the correct words and approximate words.

RESULTS

Table 79 gives the means of the correct words at six age levels
for the spastics, athetoids and tension athetoids. Table 80 gives
the means for the approximated words.

When an analysis of variance was done on the words correctly
pronounced by spastics, athetoids and tension athetoids, it was
found that the F value for the three groups was less than 1. Thus,
statistically the differences among them are not significant. The age
factor was significant, but the interest here is on group rather than
age differences. The same situation holds true for the three groups
in respect to words approximately pronounced. The F value for
the differences again is less than 1, indicating that there is no
evidence to reject the null hypothesis.

Thus, on the basis of either an analysis of phonetic elements or

TABLE 80
Mean Approximated Words of Children with Cerebral Palsy

CA	Spastic		Athetoid		Tension Athetoid	
	N	Mean	N	Mean	N	Mean
1–2	22	3.1	6	6.8	6	2.7
3–4	40	9.9	27	4.1	8	4.0
5–6	26	13.4	25	12.0	14	8.4
7–8	23	11.7	10	12.6	11	10.6
9–10	9	13.6	10	14.0	9	13.6
11–12	8	19.1	8	10.6	4	14.0

words, either spoken correctly or approximately, there appears to be no stastistical evidence for the hypothesis that differences exist in the vocabularies of spastics, athetoids and tension athetoids. The data also show that age is a factor. Cerebral palsied children use about twice as many approximate as correct pronounciations.

Chapter 42

A Comparison of the Vocabularies of Use and of Understanding

THE PURPOSE OF this study was to determine the extent of the vocabulary of expression or use and of the vocabulary of comprehension by cerebral palsied children from 6 to 17 years of age.

PROCEDURE

The vocabulary of use in this study is defined as the group of words actually verbalized. The vocabulary of understanding is defined as those words recognized in a picture vocabulary test. The Peabody Vocabulary Test was used to measure the children's vocabulary of understanding or comprehension. The vocabulary of use was determined by instructing the subjects to describe familiar scenes in three photographs.

From a file of several hundred pictures depicting cerebral palsied children in various scenes and situations, thirteen were selected by the experimenter. The thirteen pictures were examined and judged by ten staff members of the Institute of Logopedics with instruction to arrange them in the order of attractiveness to cerebral palsied children—in other words, to rate them according to the degree in which this type of child might identify with the scene in the picture. The judges were asked to use the following specific criteria on which to base their selections: (1) the theme of the picture should be within the experience of the cerebral palsied child, (2) the picture should be clear, (3) it should not be overcrowded or cluttered and (4) it should give an impression of some degree of activity. The ratings were tallied and the three pictures which scored highest were selected for presentation to the subjects as stimuli to elicit their verbalizations.

The photographs were 8 by 10 inches in size. One of them showed a spastic girl seated on a bench about to throw a ball. An-

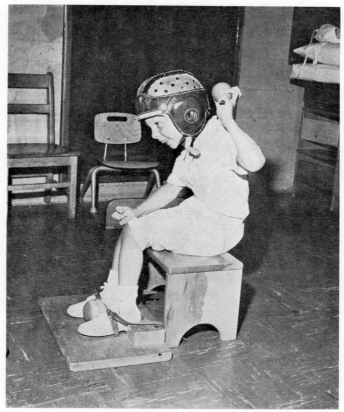

Figure 1

other was a scene including a Christmas tree with Santa Claus passing out presents to a boy in a wheelchair and to a girl seated on his lap. The third photograph was of a clown entertaining a group of cerebral palsied children. The pictures were shown without facial patches (see Figs. 1, 2 and 3).

Instructions to the Child

The tester lays out the pictures before the child and says, "Here are three pictures of children. I want you to look them over and tell me what you see in each picture; what is in it, who is in it and what are they doing. Which one do you want to tell about first?"

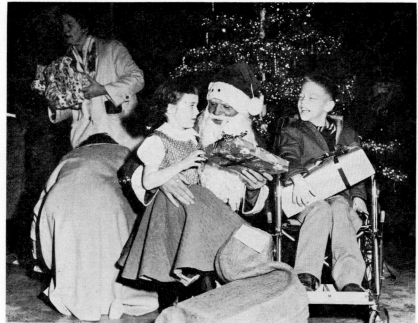

Figure 2

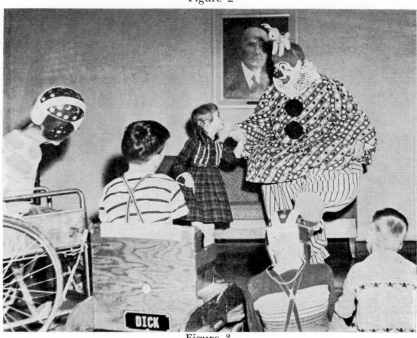

Figure 3

The tester urges the child if he hesitates in the course of his description by saying, "What else?" or "Tell me more." When the subject is finished with the first picture, he is asked to select one of the two remaining pictures and then the third until he ends his description. The subjects' responses were recorded on tape. The response period of the subject varied from two to five minutes.

RESULTS

Reliability of the Observer

Two observers experienced in working with and handling cerebral palsied children listened to the tape utterances of fifty children in response to the three pictures. Each observer independently counted the words recorded on the tape. The following rules for counting the number of words uttered are found in Appendix III in Templin's *Certain Language Skills in Children* (1957) : (1) Contractions of subject and predicate like "it's" and "we're" are counted as two words. (2) Contractions of the verb and the negative such as "don't" are counted as one word. (3) Each part of a verbal combination is counted as a separate word; thus, "have been playing" is counted as three words. (4) Hyphenated and compound nouns are one word. (5) Expressions which function as a unit were counted as one word, thus "all right" was counted as one word.

One observer heard and recorded independently 4,436 words. The other recorded 4.794 words. The precent of agreement was 92.5. The following tabulation gives the distribution of agreements. The F column gives the number of cases in the categories.

% Agreement	F
100	4
90–99	26
80–89	14
70–79	6
Mean = 92.5	50

RESULTS

The results of the investigation were concerned with the following problems: sex differences, the correlation between the vocabulary of use and understanding, the correlations between each of the two vocabularies and the chronological age, the mental age, the IQ and the frequency of parts of speech used by the cerebral palsied children. The results are reported using coefficients of correlation and analyses of variance.

The Effect of Sex

In order to determine if the scores of boys and girls belong to the same population of scores a two-by-two analysis of variance was done. Table 81 gives the means and standard deviations of both vocabularies for forty-four boys and forty-seven girls.

It is apparent from the table that the vocabulary of use by cerebral palsied children lags behind the vocabulary of understanding. The variances are somewhat heterogeneous. In order to determine if sex differences are present and also if the differences between the means of the two vocabularies are significant a two-way analysis of variance was done.

Interaction is not present and differences between the two types of vocabularies are significant at the .001 level. Since sex differences are not significant the scores of the boys and girls may be combined and treated together in subsequent analyses.

Correlation of Vocabularies of Use and Understanding

The analysis of variance presented evidence for a significant difference between the means of the two vocabularies. However, the question may be asked if there is any association at all between them and the degree of predictive efficiency. For this purpose the scores of the two vocabularies were correlated. The cofficient of correlation was .55, significant at the .01 level. However, establishing the significances of a coefficient of correlation does not mean it is a useful predictor. In order to evaluate a correlation its coefficient of determination (r^2) and its pre-

TABLE 81

Sex Differences, Means and Standard Deviations of Vocabulary of Use and of Understanding by Cerebral Palsied Children

	Male			Female		
	N	M	σ	N	M	σ
Use	44	46.8	23.4	47	37.8	20.3
Understanding	44	77.2	18.0	47	71.5	21.9

dictive efficiency, ε,* should be stated. Squaring the r gives the proportion of the variance of one factor which is accounted for by the other. Thus $r^2 = .30$ which means that 30% of the variance of one vocabulary is associated with the other. Thus the coefficient of nondetermination amounts to 70%. The coefficient of forecasting efficiency for an r of .55 is only 17%. Whereas there is a relationship of the vocabulary of use to the vocabulary of understanding, and ε of 17% suggests than an r of .55 is not a very strong predictor.

Parts of Speech

The mean frequencies of parts of speech present in the vocabulary of use are given in the next table.

The table indicates that nouns predominate in the vocabulary of use as measured by the method employed. Adjectives are next in frequency followed by prepositions, verbs, gerunds and pronouns.

Relation to Chronological Age

The relation of the vocabulary of understanding and of use to chronological age was determined. The coefficient of correlation of the vocabulary of understanding and chronological age was $r = .80$ which was significant at the .01 level. The coefficient of determination was $r^2 = .64$. The coefficient of predictive efficiency for an r of .80 is 40%.

---

*ε $= 1 - \sqrt{1 - r^2}$

TABLE 82

Mean Frequency of Parts of Speech Used by Cerebral Palsied Children

	M	Range*
Nouns	14.5	2 – 40
Pronouns	3.4	0 – 9
Adjectives	7.2	0 – 26
Verbs	4.4	0 – 17
Adverbs	1.7	0 – 6
Prepositions	4.5	0 – 13
Conjunctions	0.9	0 – 3
Gerunds	4.1	0 – 9
Interjections	0.3	0 – 1

*With these data the range gives a better statement of the distribution than the standard deviation.

The coefficient of correlation of the vocabulary of use and chronological age was $r = .37$, significant at the .01 level. The predictive efficiency of this r is 14%. It would appear that chronological age is a better predictor with the vocabulary of understanding than with that of use.

TRENDS. In order to determine trends in the data, tables have been constructed for chronological age and for mental age. The means and standard deviations of the vocabularies of use and understanding of four chronological age groups of cerebral palsied children were determined. The vocabulary of use increased from 21.9 ± 13.0 at the youngest age to 55.9 ± 22.9 at sixteen years. The vocabulary of understanding increased from 53.7 ± 10.9 to 101.0 ± 11.5. Both trends are statistically significant. The means of the vocabulary of understanding at each chronological age level are greater than those for use.

Relation to Mental Age

The coefficient of correlation of the vocabulary of understanding and mental age could not be determined because the mental ages were derived from a previous administration of the Peabody test. The vocabulary scores of understanding also were derived from a later administration of this test. Thus coefficients of correlation of the vocabulary of understanding with mental age and with IQ would be spuriously high.

The coefficient of correlation of the vocabulary of use, however, and mental age was $r = .55$. The significance was at the .01 level. The coefficient of determination is 30%. This means there is an absence of association of 70%. In spite of a correlation of only .55, it is still possible that the mental age trend may be significant.

TREND. The means of the vocabulary of use for five mental age levels show a trend from 22.0 ± 14.5 to 59.9 ± 20.3 for the younger to the older mental age level. The probability value of the trend in vocabulary of use with mental age lies at the .001 level.

Relation to IQ

The coefficient of correlation of the vocabulary of use and the IQ was $r = .07$. This value is not significant.

Ratio of the Two Vocabularies

The total number of words in the vocabulary of use was 3,740. For the vocabulary of understanding it was 6,666. The ratio of the vocabulary of understanding to that of use is 1.78.

SUMMARY

This study is a comparison of the vocabulary of use and understanding of ninety-one cerebral palsied children from 5 to 17 years of age. The children were from the provinces of Manitoba and Ontario, Canada. The Peabody Picture Vocabulary Test was used to measure the vocabulary of understanding and three selected photographs of familiar scenes served as stimuli to evoke verbalizations of the subjects. The vocabularies of use were taped. Observer agreement in reading the tape was 92.5%.

Sex differences between the means of the vocabularies of use and understanding were not present. The coefficient of correlation between the two vocabularies was $r = .55$, significant at the .01 level. Thus an association exists amounting to 30%. This yields a coefficient of predictive efficiency of .17. The coefficient of correlation of chronological age and the vocabulary of understanding was .80. With the vocabulary of use it was .37. An analysis of variance for trend with chronological age was significant and the difference between the age means for the two vocabularies was significantly in favor of the understanding vocabulary. The coefficient of correlation of the vocabulary of use and mental age was $r = .55$, significant at the .01 level. The trend of this vocabulary with mental age was significant. The coefficient of correlation of the vocabulary of use and the IQ was $r = .07$.

The best predictor among these correlations is between chronological age and the vocabulary of understanding. The forecasting efficiency is 17%. This however is not a very efficient predictor. The forecasting efficiency of chronological age and the vocabulary of use is 14%. The coefficient of correlation of mental age and the vocabulary of use yielded an $r = 17\%$. The vocabulary of understanding exceeds that of use by about 1.78 to 1.00. The mean values of the parts of speech in the vocabulary of use were reported.

Chapter 43

Vocabulary Ability of Two Samples of Cerebral Palsied Children

IN A PREVIOUS SECTION it was reported that severely involved cerebral palsied children made a somewhat better average score on the Peabody Picture Vocabulary Test than mildly and moderately involved children. This finding obviously contravenes a common sense view. An analysis of variance, however, revealed that the tendency was only apparent and was not statistically significant. The purpose of the present investigation was to replicate and check the earlier study.

PROCEDURE

The Peabody Vocabulary Test was administered first to eighty-six cerebral palsied children ranging in age from 6 to 17 years. The children were from states in the northwestern part of the country and from Hawaii. In the second sample were included 103 cerebral palsied children of comparable range from the Canadian provinces of Manitoba and Ontario.

RESULTS

In Table 83 are found the means and standard deviations of the two samples of mildly, moderately and severely involved cerebral palsied children.

As previously reported, it turned out that the differences among

TABLE 83
Peabody Picture Vocabulary Test (Form X)
Means and Standard Deviations of Vocabulary Scores by Degree of Cerebral Palsy

	Sample 1			Sample 2		
Diagnosis	N	M	σ	N	M	σ
Mild	34	68.5	17.2	25	71.1	14.8
Moderate	30	71.9	14.0	43	75.0	22.6
Severe	22	77.4	20.7	35	72.6	19.6

222

the means of sample 1 were not significant. However, a trend was apparent for the mean scores to increase from the mild to the severe groups. Accordingly a second sample of data was secured to learn if it would exhibit a similar trend in which the severe cases would exceed the mild and moderate.

Inspection of the means of the second sample indicates that the trend is not present.

A two-by-three analysis of variance was done on the means of Table 83 affording evidence that the null hypothesis may be accepted. Since the variances in the two samples of the moderates are not homogeneous, a modified t was used instead of an analysis of variance. The analysis failed to yield significance.

SUMMARY

In a previous study a trend in the mean vocabulary scores of eighty-six mild, moderate and severe cases of cerebral palsy was exhibited supposedly indicating that children with severe involvement were superior to moderate and mild cases. An analysis of variance, however, indicated that the trend was not significant statistically. In order to provide a further check on this result the study was replicated using 103 cerebral palsied cases. A 2 by 3 analysis of variance involving both samples was performed providing evidence that neither the difference between the samples was significant nor that the differences among the degrees of involvement were significant. Interaction was not present in the data.

In this investigation as well as in a study of sound discrimination and an investigation of abstraction by cerebral palsied children, no significant differences among the means of the mild, moderate and severe cases were found. These findings are all in contrast to those obtained with an articulation test where severely involved children are definitely inferior to the mild and moderate cases.

Chapter 44

The Relation of Vocabularies of Use and Understanding to Several Variables

THIS STUDY IS concerned with the relation of the vocabularies of use and understanding to the type, extent and degree of cerebral palsy. It also considers their relation to therapists' ratings of general speech and language ability of the subjects.

PROCEDURE

Ninety-one cerebral palsied children in Canada ranging in age from 5 to 17 years were subjects in the investigation. Pertinent and detailed information about them is found in the Appendix.

The children were administered the Peabody Picture Vocabulary Test, Form A. The vocabulary score was taken as a measure of the vocabulary of understanding. Three pictures illustrating scenes with which this type of child can identify were presented one at a time to the child with the instruction to tell what or who was in the picture and what they were doing. The number of words used by the subject constituted the score of the vocabulary of use.

RESULTS

Relation to Type of Cerebral Palsy

Table 84 provides the means and standard deviations of the vocabulary of use and of understanding by several types of cerebral palsy.

The table indicates that the vocabulary of understanding greatly exceeds that of use for each of the types of cerebral palsy. Since the means of the two groups do not form a consistent pattern, it may be suspected that interaction is present. In order to verify these observations, a two-by-three analysis of variance was run on the data. The analysis of variance indicated that interaction is not

TABLE 84
**Means and Standard Deviations of the Vocabulary of Use and of
Understanding by Types of Cerebral Palsy**

		Use		Understanding	
Type	*N*	*M*	*σ*	*M*	*σ*
Spastic	65	41.7	19.7	73.3	18.3
Athetoid	16	36.7	23.6	73.6	28.0
Others*	10	44.3	26.5	72.3	16.5

*Others includes mixed and ataxic cases.

present. It also revealed that differences among the means of the types of cerebral palsy are not significant. However, the difference between the two vocabularies for each of the types is significant at the .001 level.

Relation to Extent of Cerebral Palsy

The effect of extent of cerebral palsy on the two vocabularies is given in Table 85.

The table shows that for each category of the extent of paralysis the vocabulary of understanding exceeds that of use. An analysis of variance showed that interaction is not significant in these data. The differences among quadriplegics, hemiplegics and paraplegics are not significant. For each of these groups of cerebral palsied children the vocabulary of understanding significantly exceeds that of use.

Relation to Degree of Involvement

In Table 86 are found the data indicating the relation of degree of involvement, mild, moderate and severe to the two vocabularies.

TABLE 85
**The Effect of Extent of Cerebral Palsy on the Vocabulary of Use
and of Understanding**

		Use		Understanding	
Type	*N*	*M*	*σ*	*M*	*σ*
Quadriplegia	56	40.2	22.0	74.0	21.8
Hemiplegia	12	40.5	24.4	70.6	16.3
Paraplegia	17	43.8	18.1	70.4	19.7
Others*	6	43.2	14.5	79.3	11.0

*Others includes triplegics and monoplegics.

TABLE 86

**Means and Standard Deviations of Vocabulary of Use and of Understanding
According to Degree of Cerebral Palsy Involvement**

	Mild			Moderate			Severe		
	N	M	σ	N	M	σ	N	M	σ
Use	23	37.9	19.4	39	43.2	24.1	27	42.3	18.3
Understanding	23	68.3	17.0	39	74.9	22.8	27	74.3	18.4

For each of the three categories of degree of involvement the means of the vocabulary of understanding is larger than that for use. Inspection of the means of the table suggests that the similarity of pattern indicates that interaction is at a minimum. This was tested in a two-by-three analysis of variance. Interaction was found to be nonsignificant. Although the mild cases achieve a lower mean than moderates and severe cases, the degree of involvement was not a factor, but the difference of means of the two vocabularies for each degree of involvement again was highly significant.

Relation to Therapists' Rating

Seventy-five of the ninety-one cases were rated by the speech therapist on general speech and language ability. A five-point scale was employed, the ratings being very good, good, medium, poor and very poor. Very good was taken to mean normal, and very poor means barely intelligible. The remaining steps indicate the intermediate ratings. In the case of the vocabulary of use the means range from 23.3 ± 14.1 for very poor to 54.7 ± 14.4 for children rated very good. Variances are homogeneous. For the vocabulary of understanding the means were all in the lower 70's. The variances were heterogeneous. Interaction was not present and differences between the two vocabularies again were significant.

SUMMARY

This study investigated the effect of the type, extent and degree of cerebral palsy on the vocabularies of use and of understanding. It also considered the relation of vocabulary achievement by cerebral palsied children to their speech and language ratings by speech therapists. Ninety-one cerebral palsied children in Canada ranging in age from 5 to 17 years were given the Peabody Vocabulary Test in order to secure a measure of the vocabulary of understanding. The children also were asked to describe three photographs of cerebral palsied children in familiar scenes. The number of words uttered by the children constitutes the score of the vocabulary of use.

When the scores of the two vocabularies of spastic and athetoid children were compared and subjected to an analysis of variance, it was found that the difference between the means of scores of these types of children was not statistically significant. On the other hand, the difference between the two vocabularies was significantly in favor of the vocabulary of understanding.

No significant differences were present among quadriplegics, hemiplegics or paraplegics on either vocabulary. However, the superiority of vocabulary of understanding among these groups was found to be significant.

The mean scores of both vocabularies showed no significant differences in terms of the medical diagnosis of mild, moderate and severe involvement. Again the difference between the vocabularies for each of the groups was significant.

Children rated by speech therapists for general language ability as very good, good, medium, poor and very poor showed no significant differences on either vocabulary, but the difference between the two vocabularies was acceptable statistically.

Chapter 45

A Comparison of the Vocabularies of Use and of Understanding by Mentally Retarded Children

IN AN EARLIER CHAPTER a comparison was made of the vocabularies of use and of understanding of cerebral palsied children. The purpose of the present investigation was to determine the extent of the vocabulary of use and of the vocabulary of comprehension by mentally retarded children from 5 to 17 years of age.

PROCEDURE

One hundred and five mentally retarded children, sixty boys and forty-five girls were subjects in the study. The mean chronological age was 9 years, 6 months. The range was 5 to 16 years. The mean mental age was 5 years, 6 months, the range being 2 to 11 years. The children were in state hospital schools and public schools in the states of Iowa, Minnesota, Missouri, Nebraska, North and South Dakota and Wisconsin.

The Peabody Picture Vocabulary Test was utilized to measure the vocabulary of understanding. The vocabulary of use in this study is defined as the words actually verbalized. The vocabulary of use were words used by the child to describe three pictures. The responses were taped.

Reliability of the Observer

Observer reliability was reported previously. The mean percent of agreement was 92.5.

RESULTS

The results of the investigation were concerned with sex differences, the correlation between the two vocabularies, the correlation between each of the two vocabularies and chronological age, mental age and IQ.

228

TABLE 87

Sex Differences, Means and Standard Deviations of Vocabulary of Use and of Understanding by Mentally Retarded Children

	Male			*Female*		
	N	M	σ	N	M	σ
Use	60	54.0	42.7	45	45.8	29.5
Understanding	60	62.5	13.0	45	59.6	16.6

The Effect of Sex

Table 87 gives the means and standard deviations of the two vocabularies for boys and for girls.

The table shows a tendency that for mentally retarded children the vocabulary of understanding exceeds that of use. A similar finding was reported for cerebral palsied children. An analysis of variance was done to determine if sex differences are significant and also if the differences between the vocabulary means are significant. Sex differences were not significant. Vocabulary differences did not attain the .05 level of probability.

Since the difference between the vocabularies is less than 19% and larger than 5%, *t's* were run on the differences among the means of the test scores for boys and girls. When this was done the differences in the vocabularies of male mentally retarded children was not significant. For females, however, the mean of the vocabulary of understanding significantly exceeds that of use. The significance of this difference was at the .01 level.

Correlation of Vocabularies of Use and Understanding

The above analysis gives only partial support for significant overall differences between the two vocabularies for mentally retarded children. It may be interesting, on the other hand, to learn if there is any correlation at all between them. When a Pearson coefficient of correlation was calculated the *r* was .55. The coefficient of determination (r^2) is .30. This means that the variance of one vocabulary is dependent upon the variance of the other in the amount of 30%. Thus the coefficient of r = .55 does not indicate a very strong association.

Relation to Chronological Age

Coefficients of correlation were calculated for the relation of the two vocabularies to chronological age. With the vocabulary of understanding the r = .24, with the vocabulary of use it was .01. Thus with mentally retarded children the relationship with chronological age is low. On the other hand the corresponding *r's* based on the vocabulary data of cerebral palsied children were r = .80 for the vocabulary of understanding and .37 for use.

AGE TRENDS. In order to determine if there was an age trend in each of the two vocabularies, the means and standard deviations of four chronological age levels were determined. The chronological age mean for use varied irregularly from 42.2 ± 11.1 at the youngest age level to 43.5 ± 26.8 at the oldest. An analysis of variance was used to determine if the trend was significant. The F value was less than 1. The chronological age means for understanding varied from 56.3 ± 13.1 for the youngest subjects to 66.0 ± 13.2 for the oldest.

Chronological age appears not to be a factor and the difference between the vocabularies is questionable for these children. It is apparent from the above analysis that the vocabulary trend for mentally retarded children according to chronological age differs from that for cerebral palsied children. For the latter the differences for age and vocabulary are both significant, but for the mentally retarded the difference for age is not at all significant and the difference between the vocabularies hardly reaches the 5% level.

Relation to Mental Age

Mental ages of the children were taken from local records at various institutions. The most frequently used mental tests were the Peabody, the WISC and the Stanford-Binet. The coefficient of correlation of the vocabulary of use by mental age was r = .25. The corresponding correlation for cerebral palsied children was .55. The coefficient of correlation of vocabulary of understanding and mental age was not calculated because the mental ages in part were derived from the Peabody test which was also used to secure vocabulary of understanding scores. The coefficients thus would be spurious.

Data pertinent to a trend analysis of the vocabulary of use according to mental age levels were analyzed. In spite of the low overall correlation of an *r* of .25 there is a progression in the size of the means with increasing age. They vary from 26.7 ± 18.5 at the youngest age level to 69.9 ± 33.1 at the oldest. The standard deviations, however, are large, but a trend analysis was done to give some indication of the effect of mental age. The analysis reveals evidence that there is a mental age trend. The correlation coefficient of .25, however, indicates that the prediction of vocabulary of use by means of mental age is unsatisfactory for mentally retarded children. This is in contrast to the result of an analysis of mental age trend of cerebral palsied cases where the trend is of greater significance.

Relation to IQ

The vocabularies of use and of understanding correlate somewhat better with IQ. The correlation of IQ and use was .44, of IQ and understanding it was .60. Yet even here when these coefficients are evaluated, a word of caution is appropriate. When the highest correlation ($r = .60$) was selected for evaluation, the coefficient of determination (r^2) is only 36%. This is the amount of effect of the variance of one factor upon the other. Further, its coefficient of forecasting efficiency amounts to only 20%. The remaining coefficients which are smaller will yield smaller coefficients of forecasting efficiency. These are not satisfactory values.

Ratio of the Two Vocabularies

The total number of words in the vocabulary of use of retarded children was 5305. For the vocabulary of understanding it was 6415. The ratio of the vocabulary of understanding to that of use by mentally retarded children is 1.20. The comparable ratio for cerebral palsied children is 1.78.

Comparison of Mentally Retarded and Cerebral Palsied Children

Two comparisons of the scores of mentally retarded and cerebral palsied children on the vocabularies of comprehension and expression were run. In one analysis there were 105 mentally retarded children and 130 cerebral palsied subjects. Included was the mean of 318 normal children for further comparison. The results follow. For comprehension, the means of mentally retarded and cerebral palsied children were 61.1 ± 15.3 and 74.7 ± 17.6. For expression, the means of the mentally retarded children was 50.5 ± 30.3 and for the cerebral palsied children it was 72.9 ± 48.8. The means for normal children were greatly in excess of these values. Their mean for comprehension was 87.1 ± 9.6. For expression it was 170.5 ± 80.1.

These values show the striking inferiority of the handicapped to the normal child's vocabularies and the much greater scatter of their scores. It is also apparent that cerebral palsied subjects are superior to mentally retarded children in both vocabularies.

In order to make a more precise comparison, forty-nine cerebral palsied children and 105 mentally retarded children were matched by including only subjects with IQs below 80. The analysis is given in the next table.

A reading of both of the above sets of means indicates that cerebral palsied children are superior to the mentally retarded groups without cerebral palsy. This holds for both the vocabulary of comprehension and expression. It was noted that the variabilities of the two groups of children are much greater for the vocabulary of expression than of comprehension.

SUMMARY

This investigation undertook the problem of comparing the vocabulary of use and of understanding by mentally retarded children. There were 105 mentally retarded children from 5 to 16 years of age. The mean chronological age was 9 years, 6 months. The mean mental age was 5 years, 6 months and the range 2 to 11 years. The subjects were from the state hospital schools and public schools in Iowa, Minnesota, Missouri, North and South Dakota, and Wisconsin. The Peabody Vocabulary Test was used

TABLE 88

Means and Standard Deviations of Vocabularies of Comprehension and Expression by 105 Mentally Retarded Children and 49 Cerebral Palsied Children With IQs Below 80

	Comprehension			*Expression*	
	M	σ	N	M	σ
Mentally Retarded	61.1	15.3	105	50.5	38.3
Cerebral Palsied	64.6	14.3	49	62.9	44.6

to measure the vocabulary of understanding. Three selected photographs of familiar scenes served as stimuli to evoke the verbalizations of the subjects. The responses to the vocabulary of use were taped. Observer agreement in reading the tape was 92.5%.

The coefficient of correlation between the two vocabularies was $r = .55$. The difference between the means of the two vocabularies, however, was short of the 5% level with a tendency of the vocabulary of understanding to exceed use. The coefficient of correlation of chronological age and the vocabulary of understanding was .24. With the vocabulary of use it was .01. An analysis of variance for trend with chronological age was not significant. The coefficient of correlation of the vocabulary of use with mental age was .25. The trend of this vocabulary with mental age was significant at the 5% level. The correlation of IQ and vocabulary of use was .44. With the vocabulary of understanding it was .60.

Comparisons with the results of this study were made with the findings of a similar study on cerebral palsied children.

PART V
SENTENCE

The sentence is the most complex structure used in communication. It is not merely a random order of words. Words are arranged to each other in a sentence according to syntactical rules. Groups of words—like phrases and clauses, subjects and predicates—are also related to each other according to rules. The conveyance of the message depends upon the observance of the rules. Otherwise mere jargon would result. The observance of the rules or their nonobservance affects the completeness of the sentence and the clarity of the message. It has an effect on the complexity of the sentence, its structure and style, its length and its intelligibility. An approach to the problem of sentence mastery by cerebral palsied and retarded children can be made by investigating the number and length of sentences in the speech of these children.

Chapter 46

Length of Declarative Sentences

IN A PREVIOUS STUDY a comparison of the vocabularies of use and of understanding by ninety-one cerebral palsied children was reported. The responses of the subjects to the test of use or expression provided a body of data which was available for the present study. The type of sentence in this test situation turned out to be exclusively the declarative type of utterance. Sixty-six of the subjects responded to the test with both complete and incomplete sentences. The remaining cases responded with only complete sentences and others with only incomplete utterances. These cases were not included in the present analysis. Thus sixty-six children had scores on both types of declarative utterances. These data were used in the present study.

The terms "complete sentence" and "incomplete sentence" are capable of different interpretations. Accordingly it is necessary to define them as they are used in this investigation. Recent linguistic theorists advocate the abandonment of the distinction. This view assumes that we express ourselves in "chunks of talk" rather than in well-constructed sentences. It states that a sentence is a free utterance, minimum or expanded—that is, that it is not included in any larger structure by means of any grammatical device (Fries, 1952).

The conventional view, on the other hand, is that a complete sentence is a meaningful word assembly exhibiting a subject-predicate structure with appropriate modifiers. The terms "subject" and "predicate" are defined in the conventional textbook fashion. An incomplete sentence then is a fragmented utterance in which either a subject or predicate or both are omitted. The data of the study may be treated in terms of either of these approaches. The analysis here will be made according to the definition of a sentence as a meaningful unit containing a subject and a predicate. The aim is to learn how well cerebral palsied children handle the subject-predicate relation in their speech and to determine the length of their declarative utterances.

The specific purpose of this study then is twofold: (1) to determine the number of complete and incomplete declarative sentences in the expressions of cerebral palsied children and (2) to determine the number of words used by these children in both complete and incomplete utterances.

PROCEDURE

A group of sixty-six cerebral palsied children, thirty-three boys and thirty-three girls when tested responded both with complete and incomplete sentences. They range in age from 5 years, 7 months, to 16 years, 1 month. The average age was 12 years, 6 months. The mental age range was from 4 to 18 years with a mean of 10 years, 5 months. The subjects were from the provinces of Manitoba and Ontario, Canada.

A three picture test designed to elicit the vocabulary of expression or use was administered to the children. The responses were taped and the sentences were classified into two groups according to their structural completeness and also according to sex. A two-way model was the statistical design applied to the data.

The analysis was done in two parts. The first considered the number of complete and incomplete sentences, the second was concerned with length of the utterance—that is, the number of words in each type of sentence.

RESULTS
Part I

In this section the number of complete and incomplete declarative sentences in the speech of these children was analyzed. Table 89 gives the means and standard deviations.

TABLE 89
Means and Standard Deviations of Number of Complete and Incomplete Declarative Sentences of Cerebral Palsied Boys and Girls

	Complete			Incomplete		
	N	M	σ	N	M	σ
Boys	33	11.5	6.9	33	7.2	4.2
Girls	33	7.8	6.4	33	5.5	3.5

The table reveals that the means of the complete sentences for both boys and girls exceed those of the incomplete sentences and that on both types of expression the means of the boys are greater than those of the girls. In order to determine if the differences among the means are significant, a mixed type of analysis of variance was done. Interaction was found to be less than 1 and thus not significant. The difference between the means of the numbers of complete and incomplete sentences was significant at the .025 level in favor of complete sentences. Boys were superior to girls (p = .05). This is an exceptional instance in which a significant sex difference occurs.

Part II

The second section of this study is concerned with the length of declarative sentences—that is, the number of words used by cerebral palsied children in complete and incomplete utterances. In order to determine the number of words per sentence, the total number for each subject was divided by the number of sentences. Thus a child who responded with four sentences and a total of twenty words received a score of 5.0. One child who expressed himself in five sentences and a total of thirty-five words received a score of 7.0. The measure then is the mean number of words per sentence per subject. Table 90 gives the means and standard deviations for the complete and incomplete sentences for boys and girls.

The table shows that the means of the length of the boys' complete sentences is larger than their incomplete utterances. A similar situation holds for the girls. In order to learn if the differences among the means of the table are statistically significant a two-by-two analysis of variance was run on the data.

Interaction was found not to be significant. Interestingly with

TABLE 90
Means and Standard Deviations of Mean Number of Words per Declarative Sentence per Cerebral Palsied Subject

	Complete			Incomplete		
	N	M	σ	N	M	σ
Boys	33	7.5	3.5	33	4.5	2.2
Girls	33	6.8	2.6	33	4.0	1.8

the measure of words per sentence per subject sex differences were not significant. This is consistent with the general results in this problem. The difference between the number of words of complete and incomplete sentences were significant at the .001 level. This means that cerebral palsied children are capable of using complete sentences more frequently than incomplete utterances.

SUMMARY

A three picture vocabulary test was administered to sixty-six cerebral palsied children. The resulting data were categorized into complete and incomplete declarative sentences according to sex. The analysis was in two parts: (1) the number of both kinds of sentences by boys and girls, and (2) the length of both kinds of sentences by sex. It was found that the number of complete declarative sentences was greater than that of incomplete sentences and that the mean for boys on the two types of sentences significantly exceeded that of girls. Regarding the length of sentences, it was found that the mean number of words per sentence was significantly larger for the complete than for the incomplete utterances. Sex differences in the mean number of words per sentence were not apparent. This study was replicated using twenty-two boys and twenty-two girls. Similar results were obtained.

In view of the large standard deviations of the means of the number of complete and incomplete sentences, this measure is less reliable than that of the number of words per sentence per subject.

Chapter 47

Number and Length of Sentences in the Language of Mentally Retarded Children

THE AIM OF this investigation was to determine the number of complete and incomplete sentences in the utterances of mentally retarded children and to determine the length of complete and incomplete sentences in terms of the number of words per sentence used by these children. The definitions of complete and incomplete sentences are found in a previous study. The term "mental retardation" is used here as defined in the modifications in the *Manual on Terminology and Classification in Mental Retardation.* "Mental retardation refers to subaverage general intellectual function which originates during the developmental period and is associated with impairment in adaptive behavior" (Heber, 1961, p. 499). The actual levels of deviation extend from borderline to profound. The corresponding range in IQs extends from 80 to 25.

PROCEDURE

A group of 105 mentally retarded children were tested with three pictures. Of these, sixty—thirty boys and thirty girls—responded with both complete and incomplete sentences. The chronological ages of the sixty children ranged from 5 years, 8 months, to 15 years, 5 months. The mean was 9 years, 8 months. The mental ages ranged from 3 years, 8 months, to 10 years, the mean being 5 years, 8 months. The IQs ranged from 39 to 85. The mean IQ was 62. The subjects were from state hospital schools and special classes in public schools in several North Central States.

A three picture test, previously described, was administered to the children with instructions to tell what they saw in each picture, who were in it and what they were doing. The responses

241

were recorded on tape. The reliability of the three picture test was found to be adequate with speech handicapped children. With a group of mentally retarded children r = .82 and with cerebral palsied children r = .96.

The sentences were classified according to their structural completeness and according to sex. The number of sentences therefore was determined in terms of complete and incomplete sentences of boys and girls. Likewise the number of words per sentence per subject was calculated in terms of complete and incomplete sentences of boys and girls. Using two observers to determine the reliability of determining the number of words in sentences, the percent of agreement amounted to 97.5.

The report is divided into two parts. The first part considers the number of complete and incomplete sentences. The second part deals with the number of words per sentence in each type of utterance.

RESULTS

Part I

In this section the number of complete and incomplete sentences in the speech of the mentally retarded children was analyzed. The data are given in Table 91.

The table indicates that there may be a tendency for the means of the boys to exceed those of the girls. The standard deviations are about the same indicating homogeneity of variances. However, they are excessive, suggesting that the differences among the means may be inconclusive. A mixed type of analysis of variance was applied to the data. The results are presented in Table 92.

The analysis of variance reveals that interaction is not present. Neither the differences between the means of the sexes nor between the means of the types of sentences achieve significance.

TABLE 91
Means and Standard Deviations of Number of Complete and Incomplete Sentences of Mentally Retarded Boys and Girls

	Complete			Incomplete		
	N	M	σ	N	M	σ
Boys	30	7.0	5.3	30	6.2	6.2
Girls	30	5.5	5.5	30	4.7	5.1

TABLE 92
Summary of Complete and Incomplete Sentences by Sex of
Mentally Retarded Subjects

Source	df	SS	MS	F	p
Between Subjects	59	1108			
A (Sex)	1	69	69.0	3.85	.10
Subjects within Groups	58	1039	17.9		
Within Subjects	60	1073			
B (Sentences)	1	19	19.0	1.04	.30
AB	1	0	0.0	< 1	
B X Subj. Within	58	1054	18.2		

The inference then may be entertained that mentally retarded children express themselves with equal frequency in complete and incomplete sentences. Comparison of mean values of this table with those of Table 86 shows that cerebral palsied children are superior to mentally retarded children in number of sentences.

Part II

This part of the study deals with the length of sentences of mentally retarded children. The measure is the number of words per sentence per subject. The data are presented in Table 93.

TABLE 93
The Means and Standard Deviations of Number of Words per
Sentence per Mentally Retarded Subject

	Complete			Incomplete		
	N	M	σ	N	M	σ
Boys	30	6.7	1.6	30	6.4	1.6
Girls	30	6.5	1.7	30	5.5	1.7

It may be noted that the four means are rather close and that the standard deviations indicate homogeneity of variance. The following summary table should reveal the presence of significant differences if any exist in the data.

It is evident from the analysis of variance that interaction is not significant. The sex factor is significant at the 5% level, indicating that boys are superior to girls. Complete sentences exceeded incomplete utterances. The next step is to apply t-tests to discover where the significant differences lie.

TABLE 94
**Summary of Number of Words per Sentence Complete and Incomplete
by Sex of Mentally Retarded Subjects**

Source	df	SS	MS	F	p
Between Subjects	59	106			
A (Sex)	1	8	8.00	4.73	.05
Subj. within Groups	58	98	1.69		
Within Subjects	60	204			
B (Words per Sentence)	1	13	13.00	4.01	.05
AB	1	3	3.00	< 1	
B x Subj. Within	58	188	3.24		

The critical difference at the 5% level is 0.9. The starred values in the table of differences reveal which are significant.

Three comparisons equal or exceed the critical difference: (1) the difference between the means of the number of words per sentence of the boys complete and the girls incomplete utterances, (2) the difference between the number of words per sentence of the boys incomplete and the girls incomplete utterances and (3) the difference between the means of the number of words per sentence of the girls complete and incomplete utterances.

Comparison of Mentally Retarded and Cerebral Palsied Children

The sixty retarded children who responded with both structurally complete and incomplete sentences were compared with the forty-four cerebral palsied children who likewise responded with complete and incomplete sentences. The groups were matched on chronological age. The mean age of the mentally retarded children was 9 years, 8 months. The mean age of the cerebral palsied children was 10 years, 6 months. The chronological

TABLE 95
**Significance of Differences Among Means: Number of Words per Sentence
with Mentally Retarded Subjects**

		A2	A3	A4
A1 = 6.7				
A2 = 6.4	A1	0.3	.02	1.2*
A3 = 6.5	A2		.01	0.9*
A4 = 5.5				1.0*

TABLE 96

Means and Standard Deviations of Number of Complete and Incomplete Sentences of Mentally Retarded and Cerebral Palsied Subjects

	Complete			Incomplete	
	M	σ	N	M	σ
Mentally Retarded	6.3	5.4	60	5.5	5.1
Cerebral Palsied	6.9	5.1	44	5.3	2.8

age range for the mentally retarded children was 6 to 15 years and for the cerebral palsied children it was 7 to 15 years.

Two types of comparisons were made. The first considered the scores of the two groups on the number of complete and incomplete sentences. The results are presented in the next table.

By inspection it is obvious that the difference between the two groups is slight both for structurally complete and incomplete sentences.

The second comparison is in terms of the length of sentences —that is, the number of words per sentence per subject. The next table gives the results of the analysis.

The table indicated that the two groups achieve about the same mean score on words per sentence per subject on the two types of utterances.

A replication of both sets of analyses yielded similar relationships. Thus it is reasonable to infer that mentally retarded and cerebral palsied children are quite similar in regard to the number and the length of sentences.

SUMMARY

Sixty mentally retarded children, 5 years, 8 months, to 15 years, 5 months, were administered a test consisting of three pictures with instructions to tell everything they could see in them. The responses were taped and the data were categorized in two ways:

TABLE 97

Means and Standard Deviations of Number of Words per Sentence per Subject

	Complete			Incomplete	
	M	σ	N	M	σ
Mentally Retarded	6.5	1.6	60	5.9	1.7
Cerebral Palsied	6.9	1.3	44	5.2	1.7

(1) number of complete and incomplete sentences of boys and girls and (2) number of words per sentence of boys and girls.

Differences between the means of number of complete and incomplete sentences did not attain significance. Sex differences were not present. The differences between the means of the number of words per sentence of boys' and girls' complete sentences failed to attain significance. The difference between the means of the number of words per sentence of boys and girls incomplete sentences was significant at the .05 level. Mentally retarded children and cerebral palsied children show little difference in sentence mastery.

Of the two measures used in these studies of the sentence, the number of words per sentence per subject is the more reliable.

This then concludes the discussion of the construct of the sentence. The next analysis will concern immediate memory span, a necessary condition of the communicative process.

PART VI

MEMORY SPAN

A cognitive function which enters pervasively into the communicative process is memory. In face-to-face communication, immediate memory span especially is an indispensable ability for the expression and reception of a message. Without it, a condition of agnosia exists. The studies which follow deal with this cognitive problem.

Chapter 48

Immediate Memory Span of Mentally Retarded Children

IN THIS INVESTIGATION the immediate memory span of retarded children without cerebral palsy combined with that of cerebral palsied children with mental retardation is compared with the immediate memory span of normal children in elementary grades.

The immediate memory span test is in three parts. One is the Wet Fall Test from the Stanford-Binet Intelligence Scale (Terman & Merrill, 1960). A second one is the Digit Span Test from the Wechsler Intelligence Scale for Children (Wechsler, 1946). The third was developed by Korst and Irwin (1968) and is entitled the Lost Boy Test. It tells what a boy should do when lost. The subjects were required to repeat the stories. The responses were taped. The immediate memory span score is the total of the scores on the three subtests. (For the Lost Boy Test see Chart 15 in the Appendix.)

PROCEDURE

Since this is a developmental study, the data are arranged according to chronological and mental ages. The scores according to chronological age and according to mental age were analyzed separately. Two hundred eighty-five children ranging in two-year chronological age levels from 6 to 7 years to 12 to 16 years were included in one analysis. Two hundred fifty-seven children ranging in two-year mental age levels from 2 to 3 years to 8 to 9 years were included in the other analysis. The IQs of all the children were 75 or less. Five hundred twenty-three normal children constituted a control group. The data were gathered in several northwestern states, in several Canadian provinces and in city school systems.

TABLE 98

Immediate Memory Span According to Chronological Age Means and Standard Deviations of Combined Scores of Mentally Retarded and Cerebral Palsied Subjects

Age Level	N	M	σ
6 – 7	31	6.2	4.5
8 – 9	53	8.7	5.0
10 – 11	73	9.4	4.8
12 – 16	128	9.5	5.3

RESULTS

The means and standard deviations for the composite immediate memory span scores of the two groups according to chronological age are presented in Table 98.

The means range from 6.2 for the 6 to 7 chronological age level to 9.5 for the 12 to 16 age level. The trend in the means is statistically significant and the variances are homogeneous.

The means and standard deviations of scores of fourth, fifth, sixth and seventh grade schoolchildren are given in Table 99.

The values of Table 98 may be compared with those of Table 99. Inspection reveals that the means of the normals are about twice those of the mentally retarded children. Moreover the scores for the normals have attained a plateau whereas those of the retarded cases have attained a plateau according to chronological age at about 10 years of age.

The means and standard deviations according to mental age of the retarded children are found in Table 100. The means vary from 5.4 for the 2 to 3 mental age level to 12.7 for the 8 to 9 mental age level. The progression is statistically significant. The variances are in general homogeneous.

The trends of the means of both chronological and mental

TABLE 99

Immediate Memory Span Means and Standard Deviations of Elementary School Children

Grades	N	M	σ
Fourth	127	18.1	2.4
Fifth	140	18.3	1.5
Sixth	129	19.1	2.6
Seventh	127	19.4	2.9

TABLE 100

Immediate Memory Span According to Mental Age Means and Standard Deviations of Combined Scores of Mentally Retarded and Cerebral Palsied Children

Age Level	N	M	σ
2 – 3	50	5.4	4.6
4 – 5	71	6.0	2.8
6 – 7	97	10.8	4.4
8 – 9	39	12.7	4.6

ages are nonlinear. Immediate memory span according to mental age proceeds slowly at the lower age level, then takes a sudden spurt between the mental ages of 4 to 7, and then proceeds slowly again but does not reach an asymptote. It is apparent from the trends that the period of the spurt is a time when more intensive memory training may be warranted.

SUMMARY

An immediate memory span test consisting of a digit span test and two stories was administered to 285 mentally retarded children ranging in two-year chronological age levels from 6 to 16 years inclusive. A second analysis was made on the scores of 257 mentally retarded children in two-year mental age levels from 2 to 9 years. The IQs of all the children were 75 or below. The control group included 523 normal children. The means for both retarded groups showed a significant trend with age. The means of the normal children were about twice those of the retarded children. The distributions of the scores of the deviate children are greater than those of the normals.

Chapter 49

Verbal and Numerical Immediate Memory Spans
of Mentally Retarded Children

~~~~~~

IN THE PRECEDING CHAPTER the composite immediate
memory span of mentally retarded children without cerebral
palsy and that of mentally retarded children with cerebral palsy
was investigated. The aim of the present study was to replicate
in part and expand this investigation using mentally retarded
children without cerebral palsy as subjects. The study has several
further purposes: to determine if there are sex differences in immediate memory span; to inquire if there are age trends in the
data; to learn if there are significant differences between verbal
and numerical immediate memory spans; to compare again the
immediate memory span of retarded children with that of normal
elementary schoolchildren.

PROCEDURE

Since there are seventeen items on the Digit Span Test and
only six possible scores on the Wet Fall Test, in order to make
the verbal test more comparable with the numerical test, the
Lost Boy Test was added. The top possible score of the two verbal
subtests taken together is twelve.

The subjects were required to repeat the two stories. They
were instructed to reproduce the digits vocally in the order in
which they were read to them. Responses were taped.

Preliminary Analysis

A preliminary analysis was made to accomplish two purposes:
to determine (1) if it is proper to administer the two stories as

---

Note: This study was conducted and written with the collaboration of Joseph
W. Korst.

a single verbal test and (2) if it is feasible to use the verbal and numerical tests together as a unified measuring instrument.

Regarding the first of these questions, it was found that the means of the two verbal subtests were the same and that their variances were homogeneous. Consequently, the items of the two subtests belong to the same population and could be combined and administered as a verbal immediate memory span test. The further question concerned combining the verbal and numerical scores to serve as an overall measure of immediate memory span. The mean for the former was 4.1 ± 2.1, that of the digit span test was 3.7 ± 2.5. Since the difference between the means was not significant and since the variances were homogeneous, it would appear that the verbal and the numerical subtests can be used as a single overall test. In several subsequent analyses it will be used as a single measuring instrument. For more detailed analyses the verbal and numerical parts of the test will be treated separately.

PROCEDURE

The data were collected from 231 children with IQs of 75 and below in state hospital schools for mentally retarded, in speech and rehabilitation centers, and special classes in public and parochial schools. Also tested for comparative purposes were 523 normal children in the fourth, fifth, sixth and seventh grades in a number of public and parochial schools.

It was necessary to find out if the mean ages of various IQ levels of the children were homogeneous. For this purpose their chronological ages were divided into three IQ levels: .10 to .30, .31 to .50 and .51 to .75. This procedure enables the mean ages to be compared. The means of the three chronological age levels were 11.7 ± 2.6, 11.3 ± 2.6 and 11.2 ± 2.3.

The mean chronological ages of the retarded children, then, at the three levels are quite comparable. Moreover, since the standard deviations are about the same, the variances are homogeneous. Accordingly, the chronological age variable in this study is well controlled throughout the IQ range.

It would be expected that with chronological age controlled for

TABLE 101
**Means and Standard Deviations of Mental Ages of Retarded Children
at Three IQ Levels
Immediate Memory Span Study**

IQ	N	M	σ
.10–.30	35	2.9	0.6
.31–.50	52	4.4	1.1
.51–.75	144	6.8	1.4

the three IQ levels, a trend in the means of mental ages in the three levels should be present. Table 101 shows such a trend.

At each IQ level the means of chronological ages for the two sexes are practically the same. They cluster closely around a value of 11.5 ± 2.5. The standard deviations throughout the table indicate that the variances are homogeneous. Accordingly, the data do not exhibit significant chronological age differences between the sexes in this sample of subjects.

A similar comparison in terms of mental ages is tabulated in Table 102 where an expected trend in the means of both boys and girls is apparent.

The preceding analyses make it evident that sex differences at each of three IQ levels for both chronological and mental ages are not present. Since sex differences are not significant, the scores of the two groups may be treated hereafter as belonging to the same population. A trend in the means is apparent.

RESULTS

The results of the study are divided into two parts. The first will treat the combined verbal and numerical data. The second will analyze the verbal and numerical data separately.

TABLE 102
**Means and Standard Deviations of Mental Ages of Mentally Retarded
Boys and Girls at Three IQ Levels
Immediate Memory Span Study**

	Boys			Girls		
IQ	N	M	σ	N	M	σ
.10–.30	20	2.7	0.6	15	2.7	1.4
.31–.51	26	4.5	1.1	26	4.4	1.0
.51–.75	85	6.9	1.6	59	6.9	1.2

TABLE 103
**Means and Standard Deviations of Immediate Memory Span Scores of
Mentally Retarded Children According to Mental Age**

MA	N	M	σ
2 – 3	37	3.9	1.4
4 – 5	55	5.9	2.6
6 – 7	62	11.1	4.8
8 – 10	28	12.9	5.3

Part I

The first analysis of the data was concerned with possible trends in immediate memory span according to chronological age. The means of the combined verbal and numerical data are 3.5 ± 1.1 for chronological age of 6 to 7 years; 7.7 ± 3.9 for chronological age of 8 to 9 years; 8.7 ± 4.5 for chronological age of 10 to 11 years; and 8.8 ± 5.8 for chronological age of 12 to 16 years. The trend in the means of the combined data according to chronological age quite obviously is curvilinear. An asymptote is approached about the tenth year.

It may be of further interest to know if a trend exists in the memory span of mentally retarded children in terms also of mental age. The data are found in Table 103.

The table indicates that the mental age trend, like that of chronological age, is curvilinear.

A comparison may be made of the results of the present study with the corresponding findings of Chapter 48. In the present study only mentally retarded children were subjects. In the other study the subjects were a mixed group of mentally retarded children and cerebral palsied children with mental retardation. While the two investigations are not strictly comparable, some differences and similarities might be pointed out. The sets of means of immediate memory span according to chronological age of the two studies while somewhat similar are not identical. However, both arrays of means exhibit the same general curvilinear trend. In the case according to mental age the trends are also similar and the means for the various mental age levels are practically indentical. It may be further remarked that the mean memory values of normal children are about twice the mean values of the mentally retarded children. Thus in this respect the present study confirms the finding of the previous investigation.

Part II

Having presented the results of the study from the standpoint of the combined verbal and numerical immediate memory span test scores, the following analyses were concerned with a comparison of the results of the two tests taken separately.

The Effect of Sex

An initial treatment of the data in this manner is concerned with the problem of sex differences of the scores on each of the two memory tests. It was found that the differences between the means of boys and girls on verbal memory was negligible. The mean for the boys was 4.3 ± 1.5. For the girls it was 4.0 ± 1.5. In the case of numerical memory the boys' mean was 4.2 ± 3.5 and that of the girls' was 4.2 ± 1.0. In view of these values, the two sexes hereafter may be treated as belonging to the same population.

The Effect of Chronological Age

The next consideration will be in terms of chronological age in order to learn if differences between the two types of memory at each of four age levels are present.

When the verbal and numerical test means for each of four chronological age levels are compared, no significant differences were found. For both columns of means, a plateau is reached about the tenth chronological year.

TABLE 104

Means, Standard Deviations of Verbal and Numerical Immediate Memory Span of Scores of Mentally Retarded Children According to Mental Age

		Verbal		Numerical		
MA	N	M	σ	M	σ	Signif.
2 – 3	57	2.3	0.3	1.8	1.4	Yes
4 – 5	69	3.3	1.3	2.6	1.6	Yes
6 – 7	73	5.1	2.3	4.8	2.3	No
8 – 10	32	6.1	2.0	6.3	3.8	No

The Effect of Mental Age

When the two sets of test scores in terms of mental age are considered separately the results may be seen in Table 104.

The table exhibits a rather interesting finding. It indicates that from the second to the fifth mental age years verbal memory significantly exceeds numerical memory. Subsequently the difference between the means of the two types of memory are slight. Moreover, for both the verbal and the numerical immediate memory spans there is a curvilinear trend from the second to the tenth mental age.

Apparently there is some difference in the course of development of verbal and digital immediate memory span according to chronological age in contrast to mental age. In the case of the former, no differences between the types of memory show up, whereas in the case of mental age some evidence exists to indicate significant differences between the two types of immediate memory. These differences occur at early mental age levels and then fade out.

SUMMARY

An analysis of immediate verbal and numerical memory of 231 mentally retarded children from 6 to 16 years of age and 523 normal children all from nine states was undertaken with a view to determine if sex differences exist, if age trends are present and if there are significant differences between verbal and numerical memory. Another aim was to compare the immediate memory span of mentally retarded with that of normal children. It was found that sex differences were not present, that both chronological and mental age trends occur, that on the mental age criterion there was evidence at younger age levels of significant differences between the two types of memory, but according to the chronological age criterion there is little difference between the two types. The mean score of the normals was about twice the highest mean score of the mentally retarded children, confirming an earlier finding.

Chapter 50

Relations Among Measures of the Immediate Memory Span

THIS CHAPTER IS concerned with the interrelations of the scores of the three memory span tests and a comparison of the immediate memory spans of cerebral palsied and mentally retarded children.

PROCEDURE

The tests were administered to 183 mentally retarded children, 102 boys and 81 girls. The chronological age range was 6 to 16 years, the mental age range was 2 to 10 years.

RESULTS

The following analyses will be made of the data: sex differences, differences among the tests and the degree of relationship among the tests.

In Table 105 the means and standard deviations for boys and for girls of each of the three immediate memory span test scores are presented.

In order to determine if the difference among the means of the scores of the boys are significant, an analysis of variance was performed. The analysis of variance provides evidence for the

TABLE 105

Means and Standard Deviations of Scores on Three Immediate Memory Span Tests by Retarded Boys and Girls

	Boys N = 102		Girls N = 81	
Test	*M*	*σ*	*M*	*σ*
Wet Fall	2.2	1.3	1.9	1.3
Lost Boy	2.1	1.6	2.0	1.7
Digit Span	4.2	3.5	4.2	3.3
Combined	8.5	5.5	8.1	5.3

TABLE 106
t-Tests of Significance of Differences Among the Means of Three Immediate Memory Span Tests of Mentally Retarded Boys

Test	diff	df	t	p
Wet Fall & Lost Boy	0.1	101	0.49	.60
Wet Fall & Digit	2.0	101	5.30	.001
Lost Boy & Digit	2.1	101	5.40	.001

rejection of the null hypothesis. In order to determine which differences among these tests are significant, t-tests were run. The values are found in Table 106.

The table indicates that the difference between the Wet Fall Test and the Digit Span Test and between the Lost Boy Test and the Digit Span Test are significant, while those between the Wet Fall Test and the Lost Boy Test are not significant.

An analysis similar to the above was done with the test scores of girls.

Table 107 presents the results when t-tests are applied to the differences.

In the case of the girls as with boys, the significant differences are found to lie between the Wet Fall Test and the Digit Span Test and between the Lost Boy Test and the Digit Span Test. The difference between the Wet Fall Test and the Lost Boy Test are not significant.

In addition to determining where significant differences among the tests lie, it is of some interest also to learn what degree of relationship exists among the tests and to evaluate it in terms of the coefficient of determination. Table 108 gives the coefficients of correlation and the coefficients of determination (r^2).

It is apparent that the coefficients of correlation fall within a moderate range. The coefficients of determination of the values vary from 29% to 41%. When these percentages are subtracted

TABLE 107
t-Tests of Significance of Differences Among the Means of Three Immediate Span Tests of Mentally Retarded Girls

Tests	diff	df	t	p
Wet Fall & Lost Boy	0.1	80	0.42	.60
Wet Fall & Digit	2.9	80	5.87	.001
Lost Boy & Digit	2.2	80	5.31	.001

TABLE 108

Coefficients of Correlation and of Determination of Three Immediate
Memory Span Tests

N = 183			
Tests	r	r²	1−r²
Wet Fall & Lost Boy	.59	.35	65%
Wet Fall & Digit	.64	.41	59%
Lost Boy & Digit	.54	.29	71%

from 100%, they yield percentages of nondetermination. With these large percentages, evidence is provided for the uniqueness of the tests which justifies the consolidation of them for use as an instrument to measure the immediate memory span of the mentally retarded child.

Comparison of Mentally Retarded and Cerebral Palsied Subjects

Mentally retarded children and mentally retarded cerebral palsied children were given the three-part immediate memory tests. There were 144 cases of the former and 68 of the latter. The mean mental age of the mentally retarded children was 7.5 years. The mean for the cerebral palsied group was 7.0 years. The range for both groups was 2 to 10 years. Since the groups were equated for mental age, the comparison could be made in terms of chronological age levels. The means, standard deviations and differences are presented in the next table.

It is quite evident that cerebral palsied children who are mentally retarded are superior in immediate memory span to mentally retarded children without cerebral palsy.

SUMMARY

This study deals with the relations of the scores of three mem-

TABLE 109

Means, Standard Deviations and Differences Between Immediate Memory Scores of
Mentally Retarded Children and Mentally Retarded Cerebral Palsied Children

	Mentally Retarded		Cerebral Palsied			
CA	M	σ	M	σ	diff	p
6–7	3.5	1.1	7.8	1.6	4.3	.01
8–9	7.7	3.4	10.7	6.2	3.0	.05
10–11	8.7	4.5	11.1	5.3	2.4	.05
12–16	8.8	5.8	10.6	4.0	1.8	.05

ory span tests, the Wechsler Digit Span Test, the Wet Fall Test from the Stanford-Binet Scale and the Lost Boy Test. These tests were given to 102 boys and 81 girls. Sex differences were not present. The Wet Fall Test and the Lost Boy Test yielded scores the difference of whose means was not significant. The differences between the means of the Wet Fall Test and Digit Span Test and the Lost Boy Test and Digit Span Test were significant at the .001 level.

The next problem to be considered is that of manifest anxiety in speech handicapped children.

PART VII

ANXIETY

Therapists are aware that children in the testing and therapy situation may show signs of unease and anxiety. This is especially evident in the speech handicapped child. The condition may be reinforced by the child's reaction to his own speech deficiency, to the presence of a stranger, to the administrator of a test or to an unusual testing or therapy situation. Fear or anxiety is an intervening variable which may disrupt the response side of communication. It is important to know if anxiety affects the cerebral palsied and mentally retarded child.

Chapter 51

A Manifest Anxiety Scale for Use with Cerebral Palsied Children

THE AIMS OF this study are (1) to determine the reliability of a manifest anxiety scale for use with speech handicapped children, (2) to learn if cerebral palsied children are subject to greater anxiety than non–cerebral-palsied children and (3) to determine if teachers can discriminate degrees of anxiety in their pupils.

PROCEDURE

The Manifest Anxiety Scale

A scale somewhat similar to one designed by Castaneda, Mc-Candless and Palermo (1956) for use with normal children was developed for use with cerebral palsied children (Chart 15 in Appendix). It consists of twenty items judged by three speech pathologists to adequately sample the functional process of anxiety and to be suitable in content and level to the problems of the handicapped child. Foils are included to check for perseveration of responses.

The study is in three parts. The first part deals with the reliability of the scale. The second is a comparison of anxiety in cerebral palsied and retarded non–cerebral-palsied children. The third is a consideration of teachers' ability to discriminate anxiety. The test questions were asked by the experimenter. The sum of "yes" answers constitutes the subject's score.

RESULTS

Reliability of the Scale

The procedure used in this study was to divide an array of test scores of a group of subjects into odd-numbered and even-numbered subarrays according to the order in which the scale originally was administered. Seventy-four children with a variety of types of speech handicaps were given the anxiety test. The means and standard deviations of the odd-numbered and the even-numbered cases were calculated and the significance of the difference between the means was determined. The mean for the odd-numbered group was 6.3 ± 3.7; of the even-numbered group it was 6.7 ± 3.7. Since the standard deviations were the same, any difference between the groups must lie in the central tendencies. Alpha was set at .05. When the *t* statistic was calculated, it was found to be 0.45, df = 72 and p = .60, which indicates that the null hypothesis may be accepted. Accordingly, this result may be taken as evidence for the reliability of the scale. Construct validity—namely, that the items of the scale should adequately tap the process or function of manifest anxiety—was provided by the manner in which the items were judged and selected by the speech pathologists.

Matching Procedure

From the pool of seventy-four children, twenty-seven who were diagnosed as having cerebral palsy were matched with twenty-seven retarded non–cerebral-palsied children. The latter included functional cases, stutterers and aphasics. The two groups were matched on chronological age, mental age and language ability. The mean chronological age of the cerebral palsied children was 11.3 ± 3.4 years while that of the non–cerebral-palsied children was 10.0 ± 2.9 years. The difference between the means was not statistically significant. The mean mental age of the cerebral palsied children as measured by the Peabody Picture Vocabulary Test was 8.4 ± 2.7, that of the other group was 9.9 ± 3.8. This difference also was not significant.

The two language tests which were administered were two which do not involve motor ability in which the cerebral palsied children might be at a disadvantage. They were sound discrimination and abstraction tests. The means of the two groups on sound discrimination were 21.6 ± 3.2 and 20.7 ± 4.6. The difference was not significant. In the case of abstract ability the means were 19.9 ± 3.9 and 19.7 ± 4.6. Obviously the difference

TABLE 110
Means, Standard Deviations and t Value of Differences Between Manifest Anxiety Scores of Cerebral Palsied and Non–Cerebral-Palsied Children

Groups	N	M	σ	diff	df	t	p
Cerebral Palsied	27	6.7	3.6				
Non–Cerebral Palsied	27	5.0	2.4	1.7	52	1.95	.05

did not attain the .05 level of significance. In terms of these four criteria, it seems reasonable to assume that the two groups were fairly well matched.

The next section is concerned with the main aim of the study, a comparative analysis of the manifest anxiety of the two groups. The pertinent data are presented in Table 110.

It is apparent that cerebral palsied children score higher on this manifest anxiety scale than non–cerebral palsied children of the same chronological age, the same mental age and equal language ability. This is to be interpreted to mean that in their self-evaluation cerebral palsied children are probably more subject to anxiety than are non–cerebral-palsied children. That is to say, this finding holds to the extent that the children's answers to the test items are an actual reflection of their subjective experience. It is necessary then that precautions be taken to put the subject at ease in the testing situation.

One of the aims of the study was to learn if teachers or clinicians are able to discriminate degrees of anxiety in their pupils. Fifty-eight of the children also had been rated by their teachers. Ratings were according to a four-point scale of anxiety: very mild, mild, moderate and severe. The children's scale scores were assigned to these categories. The means of each rating are given in Table 111.

When an analysis of variance was done on the means of the

TABLE 111
Means and Standard Deviations of Children's Manifest Anxiety Scores According to Teachers' Ratings

Degree of Anxiety	N	M	σ
Very Mild	11	6.5	3.9
Mild	17	5.9	3.4
Moderate	14	5.8	2.7
Severe	16	6.9	2.8

table none of the differences were significant. It is rather astonishing that the teachers did not discriminate between the extreme cases of mildly anxious children and the severely anxious children.

SUMMARY

The purposes of this study were to determine the reliability of a manifest anxiety scale for use with cerebral palsied children, to determine if these children manifest greater anxiety than non–cerebral-palsied cases and to learn if teachers are able to discriminate degrees of anxiety in their pupils. When the scores of a group of seventy-four children with mixed diagnosis were divided into odd and even arrays the mean difference between them was found not to be significant. When twenty-seven cerebral palsied and twenty-seven retarded non–cerebral-palsied children were matched on chronological age, mental age and language abilities, the mean score of the former significantly exceeded the latter. It was found that teachers who rated the children on a four-point scale were unable to discriminate the degrees of anxiety of their handicapped pupils. When testing a handicapped child, it is preferable to estimate his anxiety by means of the manifest anxiety scale than to rely on the teacher's or clinician's judgment.

The next chapters will be concerned with an overall approach to language problems of the cerebral palsied and mentally retarded child.

PART VIII

LANGUAGE

The definitions of language are numerous and controversial. They vary from the statement that it expresses ideas, feelings and volitions (Wundt, 1900) to the notion that it is a device for influencing human behavior and attitudes (De Laguna, 1927). It is asserted that language embodies and determines our view of reality and of the world (Whorf, 1961). It has been defined as an arbitrary correlation between sound and meaning (Chomsky, 1964). It has been treated from an engineering standpoint in information theory as "bits" of information (Harttey, 1928). It is considered to be a system of signs with rules for their use. Some definitions are limited to the formal aspects of syntax (Carnap, 1937). They are technical and are couched in a meta-language, others are personal and practical. Some emphasize the stimulus properties of communication, others the semantic content resulting in a confusion of theories of meaning. Other definitions emphasize the response characteristics of communication—that is, the effectiveness of the message to the recipient.

It might appear that the terms "language" and "communication" may be equivalent. The disjointed and controversial nature of the definitions of language, however, makes for conceptual looseness. The term "communication," on the other hand, as it has been analyzed and defined in these pages, is a tighter and more readily applied concept. Moreover it has heuristic value. It provides opportunity and incentive for the elucidation and perhaps discovery of further variables. This consideration is important particularly in the area of communication of the speech handicapped child where our knowledge still is imperfect as the incompleteness of some of the studies in this book testifies.

Having analyzed and discussed separately various speech problems of cerebral palsied and mentally retarded children, it becomes necessary to provide an overall approach to them. Accordingly this sector of the investigation presents results of the administration of batteries of tests to samples of speech handicapped children. Analyses of the interrelations of several speech variables also will be undertaken.

Chapter 52

A Language Test

PROCEDURE

A BATTERY CONSISTING OF four subtests was administered to 107 cerebral palsied children in order to evaluate their ability to articulate, to discriminate sounds, to perform the mental function of abstracting meanings and to understand words. A second purpose was to determine the interrelations of these variables. A further aim was to study the effect of sex, of type and extent of cerebral palsy, and the relation of the scores on the test to therapists' ratings of the children's general language ability.

The Four Language Tests

The four measures consisted of a consonant articulation test, a test of discrimination of consonant sounds, an abstraction test and the Peabody Picture Vocabulary Test.

The articulation test consisted of ten difficult consonants, each in the initial, medial and final positions of words. It was originally standardized on a group of mentally retarded children and restandardized for use with cerebral palsied children. The sound discrimination test was devised in two forms for use with cerebral palsied children. Form A was used in the present study. Two forms of the abstraction test were built for use with either cerebral palsied or mentally retarded children. Form X was used in this investigation. Form A of the Peabody Picture Vocabulary Test was the fourth instrument administered to the cerebral palsied children. Although to articulate sounds is more or less a rote process, the other three tests require, in various degrees, higher mental processes.

271

TABLE 112
**Means and Standard Deviations of Language Test Battery of
Cerebral Palsied Children**

	N	M	σ
Males	58	132.6	23.7
Females	49	123.5	27.2

Observer Reliability

The agreement between two observers recording independently the responses to each of the four tests averaged about 90%.

Reliability and Validity

Each of the four subtests previously had been standardized in terms of an item analysis, test reliability and validity. The reliabilities and validities of the tests were found to be satisfactory.

RESULTS

The Effect of Sex

The first analysis is concerned with the effect of sex. The means and standard deviations for boys and girls in terms of total scores on the four tests are found in Table 112.

The variances are homogeneous. $F = 1.31$, df = 49 and 58, $p = .10$. The difference between the means of the boys and girls is not significant. Since this is the case and since the variances are homogeneous, the two groups of scores may be treated in subsequent analyses as belonging to the same population.

Scores of the Four Tests

The means and standard deviations of the scores on the four tests and the total score are presented in Table 113.

TABLE 113
**Means and Standard Deviations of Scores on the Four Tests
of Cerebral Palsied Subjects**

Test	N	M	σ
Articulation	107	20.4	8.6
Sound Discrimination	107	18.7	4.8
Abstraction	107	18.4	5.6
Vocabulary	107	70.9	15.3
Total	107	128.4	82.3

The articulation test was a short consonant test (D. Irwin, 1966). The mean articulation score of 20.4 ± 8.6 is almost identical with the score of 20.3 ± 8.7 obtained in a previous study on 114 cerebral palsied children. Likewise the mean score of 18.7 ± 4.8 for discrimination of consonants by the 107 cerebral palsied children corresponded to that of 19.0 ± 5.5 for a sample of 85 children. The mean score of 18.4 ± 5.6 on the abstract test was quite similar to 19.8 ± 5.3 on the first sample. Moreover, the mean vocabulary score was close to that of the first sample. It is 70.9 ± 15.3 as compared with 72.0 ± 16.0 for the previous sample. Thus the values of the present investigation confirm those of the earlier studies.

It will be noted that the mean of the total scores amounts to 128.4. Since there is a total of 225 items in the battery, the mean for the 107 cerebral palsied children is 57% of the possible total score (128.4/225.0).

Intercorrelations of Tests

The scores for the four subtests were intercorrelated. Also the total score of the battery was correlated with chronological age. Table 114 gives the Pearson *r*s.

The table shows that the coefficient of correlation of the total score and chronological age amounts to r = .15. This suggests that chronological age has low forecasting efficiency for language ability of cerebral palsied children as measured by this test. Moreover, chronological age correlations with the four subtests are all low.

It is seen also that articulation as measured by the short consonant test correlated low with sound discrimination, with the

TABLE 114
Intercorrelations of Subtests of a Language Examination of Cerebral Palsied Subjects

	Sound Discrimination	Abstraction	Vocabulary	CA
Articulation	.18	.26	.22	.06
Sound Discrimination		.71	.63	.37
Abstraction			.67	−.02
Vocabulary				.17
Total Score				.15

TABLE 115
**Means and Standard Deviations of Scores on a Language Test
According to Type of Cerebral Palsy**

Type	N	M	σ
Spastic	73	128.8	25.9
Athetoid	16	132.8	28.5
Mixed	13	119.2	21.5
Ataxic	3	133.7	—
Rigid	2	132.5	—

ability to abstract meanings and with vocabulary. The coefficient of correlation of sound discrimination and abstraction is .71. This is the highest value in the table. It may be accounted for by the fact that both of these behaviors involve in some degree higher mental processes. Not only is there a discriminative ability and an abstractive process involved in these responses but to a degree auditory memory is also involved since the problem required an amount of time by the child to make a choice among multiple items. The act of understanding words also is a mental process. Sound discrimination and vocabulary yield a coefficient of .67. It should be pointed out, however, that an r of .71 yields a coefficient of determination (r^2) of .50 which in turn provides an index of forecasting efficiency (ε) of about 30%. Thus the three correlations, while substantial, are only moderately useful for predictive purposes.

Effect of Type of Cerebral Palsy

Table 115 gives the pertinent data according to type of cerebral palsy.

In order to learn if the differences among the means of the spastic, athetoids and mixed cases are statistically significant an analysis of variance was done with the result that $F = 1.06$, $df = 2$ and 99, and $p = .30$. This is evidence that on this language battery spastics and athetoids do about equally well.

Effect of Degree of Involvement

When the subjects are classified according to degree of paralytic involvement the results may be seen in Table 116.

When an analysis of variance was done on the differences

TABLE 116
Means and Standard Deviations of Scores on a Language Test
According to Degree of Involvement

Degree	N	M	σ
Mild	33	131.5	23.0
Moderate	30	127.8	30.3
Severe	24	129.2	22.9
Undetermined	20	123.5	63.4

among the means of the mild, moderate and severe cases, F was less than 1.00 indicating that they are not significant.

Ratings by Speech Therapists

Each child was rated on his overall speech and language ability by the therapist in terms of a scale with five steps: very good, good, medium, poor and very poor. Very good means normal ability, very poor means a minimum of intelligibility. The results are found in Table 117.

Examination of the means indicates the presence of a trend according to the therapists' ratings. An analysis of variance was applied to learn if the trend is a significant one. Since there are only three cases rated very poor, this category was not included in the analysis. It was found that $F = 11.39$. With 3 and 96 df, $p = .001$. Thus the trend is significant.

It may be of interest to learn where the significances of difference among the therapists' ratings lie. The t value for the differences between the means of the very good rating and the good was 1.02, df $= 53$ and $p = .30$. Thus there is no significant difference between these ratings. The difference between very good and medium, however, is significant ($t = 3.08$, df $= 51$, $p = .01$). The difference between good and medium is not sig-

TABLE 117
Means and Standard Deviations of Language Test Scores of Cerebral Palsied
Subjects According to Therapists' Ratings

Ratings	N	M	σ
Very Good	22	141.8	18.7
Good	33	135.3	24.7
Medium	30	123.0	23.6
Poor	15	101.6	15.7
Very Poor	3	114.3	12.2

nificant. The difference between good and poor was significant at the .001 level and that between medium and poor was at the .005 level. The difference between the means of very good and poor was considerable, amounting to 40.2. For this difference, t = 6.65, df = 35, p = .001. Therefore in view of these analyses, not only is the general trend a significant one, but in terms of the method of extreme groups—namely, the difference between the means of very good and poor—evidence for the validity of the test as a whole is provided.

SUMMARY

A battery of four tests was administered to 107 cerebral palsied children 6 to 17 years of age. The aims of the study were (1) to evaluate the ability of these children to articulate consonants, to discriminate sounds, to perform the mental function of abstracting meanings and to understand words; (2) to determine the interrelations of the scores on the subtests; and (3) to study the effect of sex, of type and extent of cerebral palsy and the relation to therapists' ratings of the children's speech and language.

The subjects were from several states in the Southwest. Mean scores of the four subtests and of the total battery are reported. They confirm previous findings. Intercorrelations among the four tests varied from r = .18 to r = .71. The correlation of the battery with chronological age was r = .15. The correlations of all four tests with chronological age were low. The effect of sex, type of cerebral palsy and degree of involvement was negligible. There was a significant trend in the mean ratings by therapists of the general language ability of the children on a scale of very good, good, medium and poor. On the basis of the method of extreme groups there was evidence for the validity of the battery as a whole. The reliability and validities of the subtests were determined previously and were found to be acceptable.

Chapter 53

Replications and Reliability of Four Speech Tests

IN THE PREVIOUS STUDY the status of four speech tests for use with cerebral palsied children was reported. The present investigation is concerned with the replication of that study. The first group hereafter will be designated as sample 1 and the later one as sample 2. The purpose of the study is to determine the reliability of each of the four tests.

PROCEDURE

The subjects were cerebral palsied children ranging in age from 6 through 16 years of age. Sample 1 was from California, Arizona, New Mexico and Texas. There were 107 children in this group. The mean age was 10 years, 8 months. Sample 2 was from the Canadian Provinces of Saskatchewan, Alberta, and British Columbia and also from three northwestern states. One hundred thirty children constituted this sample. The mean age was 10 years, 9 months.

A replication was run on four tests: (1) a short articulation test of ten consonants (vowel sounds are not included in it on the assumption that these sounds are easier for cerebral palsied children than consonants) ; (2) a parallel form test of sound discrimination; (3) an abstraction test; and (4) the Peabody Picture Vocabulary Test.

RESULTS

Replication of the Tests

Since this is a planned comparison investigation the *t* statistic rather than the F test was used to determine significance of the difference between the means of the samples of each of the four tests.

TABLE 118

Replication of Four Speech Tests of Cerebral Palsied Subjects
Means and Standard Deviations

	Sample 1		Sample 2					
Test	*M*	*σ*	*M*	*σ*	*diff*	*df*	*t*	*p*
Articulation	20.4	8.6	20.8	7.8	0.4	235	0.22	.80
Sound Discrimination	18.7	4.8	18.8	6.0	0.1	235	1.05	.30
Abstraction	18.4	5.6	19.4	5.4	1.0	235	1.06	.30
Vocabulary	70.9	15.3	74.7	17.6	3.8	235	1.31	.20

Table 118 gives the means, the standard deviations and the significance of differences of the means of the two samples for each of the four tests.

It is quite obvious that the probability values in the last column of the table provide evidence that when the tests are replicated the results of the second sample confirm those of the first. Additional verification is afforded by results obtained from three of the tests which were administered to groups of cerebral palsied children in Hawaii and the West Coast. The data are given in Table 119.

Inspection of this table reveals that the means of each of the tests are close to the corresponding values in Table 118. If measurements from sample to sample yield consistent results, the reliability of the measure is strongly suggested.

TABLE 119

Means and Standard Deviations of Scores on Three Speech Tests of Cerebral Palsied
Children in Hawaii and on the West Coast

Test	*N*	*M*	*σ*
Sound Discrimination	85	19.0	5.5
Abstraction	85	19.5	5.3
Vocabulary	85	72.0	16.0

Chapter 54

Summary of Reliability Coefficients of Six Speech Tests for Use with Handicapped Children

~·

THE PURPOSE OF the present chapter is to bring together in one place all reliability coefficients. When using a test, the experimenter and the therapist want to know several things about its reliability. Among them are the coefficient of reliability of each of the subtests and the coefficient of the test as a whole. For a diagnostic and especially for predictive purposes, the former is the more useful measure. He also wants to know by what method the coefficients were obtained. The aim then is to present this information about the battery of speech tests.

PROCEDURE

The records of a total of 1,890 children from 6 to 16 years of age from a nationwide sample were used to determine the reliabilities of six speech tests. Of this number 318 were children in the fourth, fifth, sixth and seventh grades in a public school of a small community. The remaining number included cerebral palsied, mentally retarded, aphasic and blind children. More detailed description of the subjects tested in each of these groups may be found in the Appendix.

The following tests are included in the report: (1) an integrated articulation test; (2) a short articulation test of ten difficult consonants; (3) a parallel form test of sound discrimination; (4) a parallel form test of abstraction; (5) a test of the vocabulary of use; and (6) a test of the vocabulary of understanding. The Peabody Picture Vocabulary Test was used for the latter purpose.

Note: This study was conducted and written with the collaboration of Joseph W. Korst.

279

TABLE 120
Reliability Coefficients of an Integrated Test of Articulation

Tests	Position	Subjects	N	r	PEr	Method
Consonant	Initial	CP	265	.95	.01	Kuder-Richardson
Consonant	Medial	CP	265	.97	.01	Kuder-Richardson
Consonant	Final	CP	265	.92	.01	Kuder-Richardson
Vowel	Initial	CP	265	.89	.01	Kuder-Richardson
Vowel	Medial	CP	265	.91	.01	Kuder-Richardson
Consonant	Initial	MR	162	.91	.01	Kuder-Richardson
Consonant	Medial	MR	162	.86	.01	Kuder-Richardson
Consonant	Final	MR	162	.55	.04	Kuder-Richardson
Vowel	Initial	MR	162	.75	.02	Kuder-Richardson
Vowel	Medial	MR	162	.91	.01	Kuder-Richardson

RESULTS

Tables 120, 121 and 122 give the pertinent data. They include the names of the tests, the classification of children tested, their numbers, the correlation coefficients, their probable errors and the method used to calculate the coefficients.

Table 120 presents information about an Integrated Test of Articulation. This test was administered to 265 cerebral palsied and 162 mentally retarded children. The coefficients of reliability were calculated for consonants and vowels in the initial, medial and final positions in words.

It is apparent that the coefficients with two exceptions are in the upper eighties and the nineties.

Part 1 of Table 121 gives the coefficients of reliability of the other five tests. The methods of determining the coefficients were the Kuder-Richardson, parallel form, Hoyt and test-retest. It will be noted that a short test of difficult consonants is included in this table.

In part 2 of Table 121 are found the test-retest coefficients. The retest was administered to such children who were available from twelve to fourteen months after its original administration. The test-retest coefficients were determined for the five tests taken as a unit.

All the coefficients of reliability in the table are within the range of acceptability.

In addition to the above information, reliability coefficients of the test vocabulary of use were determined on fourth, fifth, sixth

TABLE 121
Reliability Coefficients of Five Speech Tests

1. Tests	Subjects	N	r	PEr	Method
Consonant (Short)	CP	333	.87	.01	Kuder-Richardson
Sound Discrimination	CP	260	.90	.01	Parallel Form
Sound Discrimination	MR	76	.81	.01	Kuder-Richardson
Abstract	CP	142	.95	.01	Parallel Form
Abstract	MR	97	.90	.01	Kuder-Richardson
Abstract	Blind	94	.90	.01	Kuder-Richardson
Vocab. of Use	CP	76	.93	.01	Hoyt
Vocab. of Use	CP	71	.94	.01	Hoyt
Vocab. of Use	MR	61	.82	.01	Hoyt
Vocab. of Understanding	Educable	371	.83	.01	Alternate Form
Vocab. of Understanding	Trainable	220	.84	.01	Alternate Form
Vocab. of Understanding	CP	20	.97	.01	Alternate Form
2. Five Tests	CP	31	.83	.04	Test-retest
Five Tests	Aphasic	38	.86	.03	Test-retest

and seventh grade children in a public school of a small community. Table 122 gives the coefficients.

The coefficients of reliability for the vocabulary of use of school children are slightly higher than those listed in Table 121.

In view of the results presented in the three tables it may be concluded that the tests both separately and as a whole possess substantial reliability for use with speech handicapped children ranging in age from 6 to 16 years as well as for nonhandicapped elementary schoolchildren.

SUMMARY

A series of six speech tests was constructed for use with cerebral palsied and mentally retarded children. The records of a total of 1,890 children were used to determine the coefficients of reliability of the tests. The six tests were an integrated articulation test, a short articulation test of ten difficult consonants, a test of sound

TABLE 122
Reliability of Test of Vocabulary of Use Schoolchildren

Grade	N	r	PEr	Method
Fourth	67	.95	.01	Hoyt
Fifth	84	.95	.01	Hoyt
Sixth	86	.95	.01	Hoyt
Seventh	81	.95	.01	Hoyt

discrimination, an abstraction test, a test of vocabulary of use and a test of vocabulary of understanding.

Twenty-seven of twenty-eight coefficients were acceptable. One was not. The coefficient for consonants in the final position in words was .55. The range of the twenty-seven values was .75 to .95. It was concluded that the six tests may be used reliably with speech handicapped children. The test of the vocabulary of expression was found to have adequate reliability for use with non-handicapped elementary schoolchildren.

Chapter 55

Correlations of Five Speech Tests and the WISC Verbal Scale

THIS STUDY HAS two purposes. One is to investigate and replicate the intercorrelations among the scores of five speech tests. A second aim is to determine the relationship of each of the five tests to the Verbal Scale of the Wechsler Intelligence Scale for Children. Since verbal ability is basic to both the speech tests and the WISC, it may be profitable to learn to what degree they correlate.

Although the WISC Verbal Scale is a measure of general intelligence and not specifically a speech and language test, its subtests, information, comprehension, arithmetic, similarities and vocabulary are constituted of items which are similar in nature in many respects to those of the speech tests. Moreover, they elicit comparable types of responses on the part of the testee. Due to the dependence of both sets of tests on the verbal elements there should be a substantial correlation between them. It is a purpose of this study to investigate this relationship.

However, before such a relation can be established, it is necessary to determine the intercorrelations among the five speech tests. The coefficients of correlation should indicate whether the tests constitute fairly independent variables. The evidence will be presented in part I. It is important also that the reliabilities of the speech tests should be high. They were found to range from an r of .82 to .97. When taken as a unit the coefficients of reliability of the WISC Verbal Scale is reported to be .83 for six-year-old normal children and .96 for eleven-year-old children.

Note: This study was conducted and written with the collaboration of Joseph W. Korst.

PROCEDURE

The five tests were a short consonant articulation test, a sound discrimination test, an abstract test, a test of the vocabulary of use and a test of the vocabulary of understanding. In addition the verbal part of the WISC was administered to another group of twenty-eight cerebral palsied children and fifty-two children diagnosed as aphasic. The five tests together with the WISC Verbal Scale were given to the eighty speech handicapped children.

RESULTS

The results of the study are presented in two parts. The first is concerned with the intercorrelations among five communication variables. The scores of the 130 cerebral palsied cases were used in this analysis. Included in this part of the report is a check on the results in a supplementary study of the intercorrelations of scores of forty cerebral palsied children in residence at the Institute of Logopedics. The second part is concerned with the correlations of the five tests and the WISC. These calculations were based on the scores of the eighty speech handicapped subjects.

Part I

This section deals with the intercorrelations of the scores of 130 cerebral palsied children on five speech tests. The values are given in Table 123.

In general the correlations in this table are low or moderate. They range from .08 to .67. Two correlations are somewhat more prominent. The sound discrimination test and the abstract test both involve to some degree mental or conceptual processes. Thus a moderate value of the coefficient of correlation could be ex-

TABLE 123
Interrelations of Five Speech Tests of Cerebral Palsied Children

Test	Sound. Discrim.	Abstract	Vocab. of Use	Vocab. of Underst.
			$N = 130$	
Articulation	.08	.16	.33	.24
Sound Discrimination		.67	.33	.49
Abstraction			.47	.61
Vocabulary of Use				.46

pected. The coefficient turned out to be .67. The abstract test and the test of understanding also involve somewhat similar mental processes. The coefficient of correlation is .61. It should be observed, however, that the predictive value of these coefficients is low. The coefficients of determination (r^2) of .67 is .45, and of .61 it is .37. The coefficients of nondetermination then amounted to .55 and .63. The table indicates that the coefficients of correlation of articulation and the other speech variables are not very considerable. In general the results of this analysis corroborate those presented in Chapter 53.

Part II

The following table gives the coefficients of correlations of the WISC Verbal Scale with each of the five speech tests. The WISC values are scaled scores, those of the Peabody are raw scores.

The WISC scaled scores correlate .94 with the raw scores of the Peabody (vocabulary of understanding). The coefficients for the four remaining tests with the WISC Verbal Scale range from $r = .09$ to .49. The coefficients of determination of these four tests indicate that the relationships are minimal in strength. When the five speech tests are taken as a unit and correlated with the WISC Verbal Scale, the coefficient is only .50. The coefficient of determination is .25 and the coefficient of nondetermination then is .75. This means that although both are verbal tests, 75% of the variance of the speech tests is largely independent of the variance of the WISC. To say it another way, with the exception of the vocabulary of understanding, the WISC Verbal Scale and the four other speech tests measure different aspects of the verbal per-

TABLE 124
Correlations of the WISC Verbal Test and Five Speech Tests
(80 Cerebral Palsied and Aphasic Subjects)

Tests	WISC Verbal	
	r	r^2
Articulation	.09	.008
Sound Discrimination	.45	.20
Abstraction	.49	.24
Vocabulary of Use	.40	.16
Vocabulary of Understanding (Peabody)	.94	.88
Total	.50	.25

formance of cerebral palsied children. This is a consideration when the verbal ability of the cerebral palsied child is being evaluated by the WISC Verbal Scale.

SUMMARY

Five speech tests were administered to two samples of cerebral palsied children from 6 to 17 years of age. One group included 130 children, the other included forty subjects. The five tests were consonant articulation, sound discrimination, abstraction, vocabulary of use and vocabulary of understanding. The five tests and the WISC Verbal Scale were administered to eighty speech handicapped children. The purpose of the study was to investigate the intercorrelations of the five speech tests, and to determine the relationship of each speech test and the WISC Verbal Scale. The intercorrelations were generally low, varying from r = .08 to r = .67. Sound discrimination and abstract correlated .67. This value was obtained with both groups of cerebral palsied children. The coefficient of correlation for the vocabulary of use and of understanding was .46. With a second group it was .38. With a third sample of eighty children the WISC Verbal Scale and the Vocabulary of Understanding (the Peabody Picture Vocabulary Test) gave a coefficient of .94. The remaining values ranged from .09 to .49.

Chapter 56

Regional and Sex Differences in the Language of Cerebral Palsied Children on Five Speech Tests

THIS INVESTIGATION IS an effort to learn if there are differences between the performance of cerebral palsied children in Hawaii and on the mainland on three language measures. Another aim was to discover if sex differences are present. Form A of a Sound Discrimination Test, Form X of an Abstraction Test, and Form A of the Peabody Picture Vocabulary Test were administered to the children. Descriptions of these tests, their construction and instructions for administration are found in the earlier chapters.

PROCEDURE

The subjects were eighty-six cerebral palsied children, forty-three from Hawaii and forty-three from the northwest part of the country. The children from Hawaii represented a variety of stocks. Some were pure Japanese, Chinese, and Filipinos, but there were only a few pure Hawaiian children. There was considerable racial mixture, the proportions being unknown. The mean chronological age of the children in Hawaii was 11 years, 2 months. For the children on the mainland the mean age was 11 years, 8 months. The overall age range of the two groups was 6 to 17 years. The hearing of the children was tested with an audiometer or a spondee test. The criterion was the ability to hear in a conversational setting in a quiet room. Children with hearing losses were not used in the study. The diagnoses of cerebral palsy were taken from the medical records found in the children's cumulative folders.

Note: This study was conducted and written with the collaboration of Don D. Hammill.

TABLE 125
Means and Standard Deviations of Scores on Form A of a Sound Discrimination Test of Cerebral Palsied Children According to Regions and Sex

Regions	Boys			Girls		
	N	M	σ	N	M	σ
Hawaii	24	17.3	5.3	19	17.1	3.9
Northwest	24	20.1	4.7	17	21.6	5.2

RESULTS

Sound Discrimination

The first analysis is concerned with the effect of sex and geographical regions on sound discrimination. Table 125 presents data secured by using the sound discrimination test (Form A). When an analysis of variance in a double entry table was done, it was found that neither the difference between the scores of Hawaiian and mainland children nor between the sexes were significant. The F ratio was less than 1.

Abstraction

Table 126 shows the effect of regions and sex on the abstraction scores. An analysis of variance indicated that $F < 1$. Consequently the differences among the means of Table 126 were not significant.

Vocabulary

The means and standard deviations of scores on the vocabulary of comprehension are given in Table 127. From a casual observation of the table, it is apparent that the means for vocabulary of the cerebral palsied subjects from the Northwest exceeded those from Hawaii, but the F ratio was not significant. The differences among the means for the sexes also were not significant.

In summary the differences among the means for sound dis-

TABLE 126
Means and Standard Deviations of Scores on Form X of an Abstraction Test of Cerebral Palsied Subjects According to Regions and Sex

Regions	Boys			Girls		
	N	M	σ	N	M	σ
Hawaii	25	18.4	5.4	19	19.7	4.9
Northwest	25	20.3	4.9	17	21.3	4.7

TABLE 127

Means and Standard Deviations of Scores on the Peabody Picture Vocabulary Test (Form A) of Cerebral Palsied Children According to Regions and Sex

Regions	Boys			Girls		
	N	M	σ	N	M	σ
Hawaii	25	70.1	12.6	19	69.1	13.8
Northwest	25	74.2	16.3	17	74.8	20.5

crimination, for abstraction and for vocabulary both for regions and for sex were not significant. Although the differences among the means between the scores of Hawaiian cerebral palsied subjects and those from the mainland are not significant, there was a tendency of all three language aspects for the means of the mainland subjects to exceed those of the Hawaiian subjects. The slight excess may be due to the fact that the mean age of the mainland subjects is six months greater than that of the Hawaiian children. However, in spite of the age advantage, the differences among the means were not significant.

The finding of no significant differences between cerebral palsied children in Hawaii and on the mainland regarding each of the three speech variables is consistent with similar results obtained among various regions within the United States.

SUMMARY

A sound discrimination test, an abstraction test and a vocabulary test were administered to forty-three cerebral palsied children from the northwestern part of the mainland. The children from Hawaii represented several racial mixtures. The purpose was to discover if there were regional and sex differences among the children on the three variables. It may be inferred from the analyses that sex differences were not present in these data and that there were no significant differences in the performance of the Hawaiian and mainland subjects on either of the three measures.

Chapter 57

Comparison of Scores of Cerebral Palsied, Subnormal and Normal Children on Five Speech Tests

THE PRESENT INVESTIGATION is an attempt to summarize the effects of five speech variables: articulation, sound discrimination, abstraction, the vocabulary of expression or use, and the vocabulary of comprehension or understanding. For further comparative purposes a sample of the speech of normal schoolchildren is included.

PROCEDURE

In a pool of 235 handicapped children from northern states and in three Canadian Provinces, 130 were cerebral palsied and 105 were mentally retarded or subnormal without cerebral palsy. These children were given five speech tests. From this pool a group of thirty-seven cerebral palsied children were matched with a group of thirty-seven subnormal* children on IQ and chronological age. The mean IQ score for the cerebral palsied children was 68.9, for the subnormal group it was 66.7. The difference was not significant and the variances were homogeneous. The IQs ranged from 37 to 89. The mean chronological ages for the two groups were practically the same. The mean age for the cerebral palsied cases was 12 years, 3 months, for the subnormal children it was 12 years, 1 month. The range for the former was 6 to 16 years, 10 months, for the other group it was 5 years, 8 months, to 15 years, 6 months. Thus while the grouping on the basis of IQ was comparable and the means of the ages were the same, there was some difference in the age ranges.

Note: This study was conducted and written with the collaboration of Joseph W. Korst.

*The term "subnormal" is here used to include the group of children without cerebral palsy who have IQs below 90.

TABLE 128

Means and Standard Deviations of Scores on Five Speech Tests by Cerebral Palsied, Subnormal and Normal Schoolchildren

Test	N	Cerebral Palsied M	σ	Mentally Retarded M	σ	N	Normal M	σ
Articulation	37	18.8	8.2	24.9	4.9	318	29.2	3.0
Sound Discrim.	37	18.4	6.1	14.3	7.4	318	23.7	3.0
Abstraction	37	18.8	5.4	15.3	7.8	318	24.0	80.3
Vocabulary of Use	37	60.8	43.4	62.4	39.7	318	170.5	80.3
Vocabulary of Understanding	37	74.7	17.6	66.1	15.3	318	87.1	9.5

In addition 318 schoolchildren in the fourth, fifth, sixth and seventh grades in a small town were given the five tests. Their scores are included in order to show how handicapped children in general compare with nonhandicapped children.

The five tests used in the project were a short articulation test of ten consonants, a parallel form test of sound discrimination, an abstraction test, the Peabody Picture Vocabulary Test and a vocabulary of use test.

RESULTS

The means and standard deviations of the three groups of children are presented in Table 128.

It is obvious by inspection of the table that the schoolchildren are definitely superior to the two groups of handicapped children on all five of the tests. It is hardly necessary to indicate that this situation is due to superior intelligence and training. Inclusion of the means of these children is merely to point up the great difference in speech and language ability between the handicapped and the nonhandicapped child. Since the differences are striking, the application of a significance test would be redundant.

The interest in this study concerns the differences between the means of the two handicapped groups on each of the five tests rather than the differences between the means of the tests. Accordingly, this is a planned comparison investigation and the t-test of significance for unrelated measures was used instead of an F test. The significances of the differences are set forth in Table 129.

TABLE 129

Significance of Differences Between Scores of Cerebral Palsied and Subnormal Children on Five Speech Tests

Tests	CP	MR	diff	df	t	p	Signif.
				N = 74			
Articulation	18.8	24.9	6.1	72	3.81	.001	Yes
Sound Discrim.	18.4	14.3	4.1	72	2.56	.01	Yes
Abstract	18.8	15.3	3.5	72	2.19	.05	Yes
Vocab. of Use	60.8	62.4	1.6	72	0.16	.85	No
Voc. Underst.	74.7	61.1	13.6	233	2.89	.001	Yes

It will be noted that the subnormal group is superior to the cerebral palsied children on consonant articulation. The difference between the means of the two groups is significant at the .001 level. This confirms a previous finding. For sound discrimination, however, the cerebral palsied group is superior. This is consistent with previous findings. In the case of the abstraction test the cerebral palsied children also are superior to the subnormal group. This too affords confirmation of an earlier result.

Concerning vocabulary ability a different situation was obtained. The differences of means on the vocabulary of use approaches significance.

SUMMARY

From a pool of 235 cerebral palsied and mentally retarded children two groups, one consisting of thirty-seven cerebral palsied children, the other of thirty-seven subnormal children were matched for IQ and chronological age. The mean IQ for the cerebral palsied group was 68.7, and for the subnormal group it was 66.7. The mean chronological ages were 12 years, 3 months, and 12 years, 1 month. These children were given five tests: articulation, sound discrimination, abstraction, vocabulary of use and vocabulary of understanding. In addition, 318 schoolchildren in the fourth, fifth, sixth and seventh grades were tested.

It was found that the scores of the schoolchildren were greatly in excess of those of the handicapped children. On the articulation test the mean of the subnormal group significantly exceeded the mean of the cerebral palsied group. However, the cerebral palsied children were superior to the subnormal children on sound discrimination and abstract ability. The data showed no significant differences on the vocabulary of use.

Chapter 58

Recapitulation and Discussion

SUMMARY

I N THIS CONCLUDING CHAPTER a summary of the more prominent results and implications of the studies will be made. Short rather than long tests were constructed for use with cerebral palsied and mentally retarded children because they fatigue quickly while taking long tests. Moreover, their attention spans are quite brief. The tests were concerned with problems of articulation, sound discrimination, abstraction, vocabulary, the sentence, memory span and anxiety. The reliability and validity of each test has been determined.

Consideration will first be given to results of the articulation tests. The problems which demand the greater part of the speech therapists' attention are concerned with articulation. Consequently the greater part of this investigation has been devoted to these problems. Thirteen articulation tests were employed in this project. The specific results found with these tests are summarized at the end of each chapter. To summarize them again would prove to be too detailed and impractical. However, in spite of the difficulty of giving a long test to this type of child, an effort was made to do so by administering an Integrated Articulation Test to samples of children. The information obtained with this test was typical and in the main corroborated the findings of the separate short tests. It will be timesaving to summarize the information yielded by this test.

Four of the short consonant tests and the vowel test which had been standardized separately were administered as a single test to two groups of children. There were 147 cases in one group and 118 in the other.

Although there are five subtests, they do not constitute a battery in the conventional sense of the term. A battery usually is defined as a set of different and relatively uncoordinated subtests. Thus the definition of a battery is twofold; low interrelations among the subtests and dissimilarity of content from subtest to subtest. Unlike conventional instruments, the integrated test measures only one ability—namely, articulation. It does not include items of other kinds of content such as sentence structure, vocabulary or number. All five are concerned only with phonation. Such being the case, the intercorrelations among the five parts should be high. They run from r = .84 to r = .91. The high intercorrelations therefore indicate that the five parts do not function as mere subtests in a battery. They indicate rather that the test as a whole is homogeneous or integrated in nature.

It was found with the first group of cerebral palsied cases that the means of boys and girls were identical and that the variances were homogeneous. Therefore in subsequent analyses with this test their scores were treated as belonging to the same population. Observer reliability amounted to 90%. Kuder-Richardson coefficients of reliability calculated for sounds in three positions in test words varied from r = .65 to r = .97. Parallel form reliability was r = .98. Validity determined by the extreme groups method yielded a probability value of .001. Illustrations of articulation test forms and individual record sheets may be found in the Appendix.

The effects of chronological age, mental age and IQ on the integrated test scores were negligible. The means of scores in the initial position in words was significantly higher than for the final position. Spastics were more successful with this test than were the athetoids. Paraplegics made better mean scores than quadriplegics and hemiplegics. The means of right and left hemiplegics are the same as are the standard deviations. Mild cases make almost twice the mean score of severe cases.

In order to check the results obtained with the administration of the integrated test to the first group of subjects, it was replicated with a group of children in eight other states. The analyses in terms of the usual set of criteria varified the original standardization. The status of each factor treated in the first administration was confirmed by the replication.

This test also was used to study consonant and vowel difficulties. They varied from 35% to 95% which is an acceptable distribution. It is of considerable interest to learn that the order of difficulty of sounds in the initial, medial and final positions vary decidedly. For instance, the *s* sound ranks third in the initial position, eleventh in the medial and fifth in the final position. The consonant *t* ranks nineteenth in the initial position, ninth in the medial and third in the final. The vowel *o* is sixth in the initial and tenth in the medial position.

The study of the difficulties of consonants was pursued further by making the analysis according to manner of articulation, place of articulation and voicing. Instead of presenting the results as correct responses, as was done previously, these data were analyzed in terms of percent of errors, thus making the results more meaningful to the therapist. The order of difficulty of consonants when classified according to manner of articulation varied in the initial, medial and final positions. In general the nasals are least difficult for the children. Glides and fricatives are most difficult for the children. Stops, semivowels and combinations vary among the three positions. The order of difficulty according to place of articulation also varies with position in words. There is a tendency among cerebral palsied children for voiceless consonants to be more difficult than voiced sounds.

In order to use the integrated articulation test with mentally retarded children it was necessary to restandardize it on a sample of this population. The sample consisted of 162 mentally retarded children from five states. The reliability and the validity of the test were determined satisfactorily in the usual manner. The uniqueness of the items and their discriminating power exhibited the proper relationship. The difficulties of the consonants varied from 41% to 98%. The vowel difficulties ranged from 93% to 99% which is radically restricted. A similar limited spread, it was stated earlier, occurred with cerebral palsied children. The order of difficulty for mentally retarded children, as with cerebral palsied cases, is not the same in the three positions in words.

It is apparent that in some situations a short form of the integrated articulation test is needed. This project was undertaken by the author's son (Irwin, 1966). The number of consonants in the short form was limited to ten difficult sounds. In order to determine which ten sounds should be selected, an analysis of reports in the literature was conducted. Eight reports were available. The selection of the ten consonants from these lists was based on a tally of sounds common to them.

The short test of ten difficult consonants had been constructed for use with mentally retarded children. Before using it with cerebral palsied children it was restandardized on a sample of these children. Three hundred thirty of these children from fourteen states were subjects in this project.

Observer reliability was adequate. Kuder-Richardson reliabilities were in the eighties. The coefficient of temporal stability was .87 and parallel form reliability was .85. Validity as determined by the method of extreme groups was adequate. The data of this replication thus verified those secured by the longer test.

Comparisons were made of articulation scores of cerebral palsied and mentally retarded children. The comparison was investigated in two studies, one with the test of ten difficult consonants, the other using the integrated articulation test.

In the first study four comparisons were undertaken. When a group of cerebral palsied and retarded children with IQs ranging from 25 to 50 were tested, the mean score of the retarded children significantly exceeded that of the cerebral palsied individuals. With a second group whose IQ ranged from 51 to 80, a similar situation obtained. A third comparison involved cerebral palsied children whose IQs fell between 91 to 110 and retarded children with an IQ range of 51 to 80. The means of these two groups were the same. A fourth comparison included a sample of non-afflicted children with IQs between 91 and 110. The difference was significantly in favor of the normal group. The probability was at the .001 level.

It was therefore hypothesized that as far as consonantal articulation is concerned the affliction of cerebral palsy is a factor which depresses the speech ability below that found in mental retardation. This problem was further investigated using the integrated articulation test with 265 children with cerebral palsy and 162 mentally retarded cases.

The first analysis yielded the information that the means of correct scores of mentally retarded cases significantly exceeded the mean of the cerebral palsied children thus supporting the previous study. An important finding is that for errors—that is, substitutions and omissions—the means of the cerebral palsied cases very definitely were greater than those of the mentally retarded.

A further comparison was done in terms of two IQ levels, 25 to 50 and 51 to 80. In both comparisons the correct scores for the retarded on this test also were greater than those of the cerebral palsied children. Moreover for substitutions and omissions the means of the cerebral palsied cases were significantly in excess of those for the retarded. It may be suggested then that the wider scatter in frequency of articulation errors on both tests by these children is evidence for the hypothesis that the affliction of cerebral palsy is a factor in addition to mental retardation in the speech of cerebral palsied children.

A final project was the investigation of the relation of the short test of ten difficult consonants to the longer integrated consonant test. The short test was constructed on the basis of subjective judgment. On this basis its validity appeared to be acceptable. Its empirical validity, however, remained to be investigated. This was done by correlating the scores of a group of children who took both tests. The coefficient of correlation was $r = .90$. The short test then predicts the results of the longer test with reasonable efficiency. Moreover, the mean score for the test of ten consonants was 19.4 ± 9.1. This is comparable to a mean of 20.3 ± 8.7 obtained with this test previously with another sample of children. It is evident, therefore, that both the validity and the reliability of the short test is acceptable.

Whenever economy of time and cost dictate, the shorter test may be used in place of the longer instrument. It has been found useful in several investigations in this research program.

In addition a series of tests were concerned with consonant

blends. The abilities of speech handicapped children were tested with tests of initial double blends, final double blends, final double reversed blends, and triple consonant blends. These tests originally were constructed by Templin for use with normal children. Before using them with cerebral palsied subjects they were restandardized on a sample of this type of children. A vowel test and a diphthong test also were standardized.

With the series of thirteen articulation tests, there resulted a number of consistent findings. The reliabilities of the tests are fairly high. Their validities appear to be well established. Item analyses are acceptable. Correlations with mental and chronological ages and IQ are not very strong. Articulation differences between right and left hemiplegics are not significant. Quadriplegics make lower scores than paraplegics and hemiplegics. Sex differences are absent. Spastics and athetoids do equally well articulating consonant blends. However, the mean of the spastics is significantly larger than that of athetoids in the articulation of difficult consonants. Sounds in the initial position in words are easier than in the medial or final position. The orders of difficulty of sounds in the initial, medial and final positions are not the same.

Nasal consonants are easiest in the initial position. Fricatives and glides are most difficult in all three positions. In terms of place of articulation, labials are easiest and dentals and glottals are most difficult. There is a tendency for voiceless consonants to exceed the voiced in percent of difficulty.

It appears that due to the nature of their affliction cerebral palsied children are inferior to mentally retarded children in the ability to articulate sounds.

Earlier it was suggested that communication reduced to its lowest terms is articulation and discrimination of sounds. The next discussion will deal with the latter of these two terms.

Five studies were concerned with problems of sound discrimination. The first task was to construct and standardize on cerebral palsied children parallel Forms A and B of this test. In addition, Form A was replicated on a third sample of children. Both forms were then restandardized on mentally retarded cases.

Finally comparisons were made of the status of sound discrimination of cerebral palsied and retarded children.

Form A was administered to 153 cerebral palsied children in eastern and southwestern states. An analysis of variance indicated that regional differences were not statistically significant. The means of boys and girls were alike and the variances were homogeneous. Percent of agreement between two observers amounted to 96. An item analysis showed that the mean coefficient of discriminating power of Form A was .65 and of uniqueness it was .19. The range of item difficulty varied from 36% to 80%.

The reliability of Form A was determined using a Kuder-Richardson formula. The coefficient was r = .87. The validity of the test was estimated by the method of extreme groups in three ways. Arranging the discrimination scores in six chronological age levels and applying an F test for trend, the probability value was .001. On the basis of four mental age levels the trend mean scores was significant at the .001 level also. Moreover the difference between the means of very good and very poor was significant.

The effect of position of the sound in the word was determined by applying a t statistic to the difference between the means of scores in the initial and final positions. The probability value of .001 was in favor of the initial position. The difference between the means of spastics and athetoids was not significant. This is in contrast with articulation where spastics do better than athetoids. No differences exist among quadriplegics, hemiplegics and paraplegics. This was also the situation with vowel articulation, but in consonantal articulation quadriplegics make the lowest mean score.

Using 260 cerebral palsied children, Form B of the sound discrimination test likewise was standardized. The means of boys and girls in northwestern and northern central states were similar as were the means of the two regions. The reliability of Form B as calculated by a Kuder-Richardson formula was r = .88. When the scores of Form A and Form B were correlated r = .90. Thus parallel form reliability was established. The mean discriminating power of Form B was .69 and the mean uniqueness value was .23. The proper relation between discriminating power and uniqueness of items of this test was maintained. The difficulties of the items varied from 50% to 80%, a range less satisfactory than that of Form A. On Form B, unlike Form A, there was no difference between spastics and athetoids. Right and left hemiplegics oddly again made the same score, and quadriplegics, hemiplegics and paraplegics were only slightly different on this test.

Sound discrimination tests also were administered to mentally retarded children. The data were collected on mentally retarded children in Hawaii and in several northwestern states. The coefficient of test reliability was .81. This compares favorably with an $r = .87$ found previously with this test.

Validity was established in several ways. The difference between the means of scores of educables and trainables was highly significant. Also the difference between the means of extreme groups on the Peabody Picture Vocabulary Test was significant. For a final determination of validity Form A and the Templin Sound Discrimination Test were administered to fifty-two retarded children. The coefficient of correlation was .83.

A study comparing retarded children and cerebral palsied children was undertaken. Parallel form reliability was determined by administering both forms to eighty-seven retarded cases. The coefficient of correlation was .80. Thus both the reliability and validity of these tests have ample evidence for their support. It should be noted that on the basis of these investigations the mentally retarded children are inferior to cerebral palsied children in sound discrimination while the reverse is true of articulation.

This section is concerned with the processes of abstraction and categorization. The first of three investigations dealt with the standardization of a parallel form test. A second considered the relation of several factors to abstraction. The third study investigated the possibility that the test is useful with mentally retarded children without cerebral palsy.

Two test forms were administered to two samples of children totaling 142 in number. One group was from several northeastern states, the other from the Southwest. Upon the application of an analysis of variance to the data of either form it was found that neither sex nor geographical region affected the scores differentially.

The reliability of the test was handled in two ways. A Kuder-Richardson formula yielded a coefficient of .95 for Form X and .96 for Form Y. The correlation between the scores of the two forms was .95. Observer reliability using both forms with fifty-five subjects amounted to 98%. Thus there is a 2% error in the data.

Validity likewise was established in two ways. Scores on each form were correlated with the WISC Similarities Test. With Form X the coefficient was .74, with Form Y it was r = .79. It is apparent that the evidence for both reliability and validity of this parallel form abstraction test is quite substantial.

A second study investigated the relationships between the scores of the abstraction test and a number of pertinent factors. There is no difference between the means of quadriplegics, paraplegics and hemiplegics. The means of mildly, moderately and severely involved cerebral palsied cases are about the same. The mean scores of spastics and athetoids vary only a little. Form X correlates .70 with mental age while the correlation for Form Y is .76. Correlations of both forms with chronological age are low.

Form X of the abstraction test was administered to 109 mentally retarded children in Hawaii and northwestern states. When an item analysis was completed it was found that the coefficient of discriminating power was .90, and for uniqueness it was .31. The range of item difficulty was 22% to 88%. These values compare favorably with those for cerebral palsied children of .80, .34 and a range of 42% to 83%.

It appears then that the abstraction test secured both on cerebral palsied and mentally retarded children meets the criteria for the standardization of a testing instrument.

The investigation of the word equipment of speech handicapped children include the following problems: a comparison of spastics and athetoids, a comparison of the vocabulary of use and understanding by cerebral palsied children, their relation to several factors, and a comparison of the two types of vocabularies by mentally retarded children.

The first problem attacked was the word mastery by spastics and athetoids. One hundred twenty-eight spastic, eighty-six athetoids and fifty-two tension athetoids from eight states composed the sample. Analyses were made of the data according to correct pronunciation and according to approximate pronunciation. An analysis of variance showed that a significant trend with chronological age was present. The three palsied groups did not exhibit any significant differences among their means. This result was true for both correctly and for mispronounced words. The analysis also found that cerebral palsied children use about twice as many word approximations as correct pronunciations.

A comparison was made of the vocabulary of expression and the vocabulary of comprehension. The vocabulary of comprehension was defined as those words recognized in the Peabody Picture Vocabulary Test. The vocabulary of expression was determined by recording on tape the subject's description of familiar children's scenes in several photographs. Ninety-one subjects from the provinces of Manitoba and Ontario were included in the sample.

When the scores of the vocabulary of comprehension were correlated with chronological age, r was .80. The vocabulary of expression correlated with chronological age .37. The correlation of the vocabulary of expression and mental age was .55. In spite of this moderate correlation coefficient, the mental age trend was significant. The coefficient of correlation of the vocabulary of expression and IQ was $r = .07$. The ratio of the vocabulary of comprehension to expression was 1.78.

A type of study similar to the foregoing was undertaken with mentally retarded children. One hundred five children from the North Central States were subjects. With these subjects, as with cerebral palsied cases, the vocabulary of comprehension was more extensive than that of expression, but the probability value is short of the .05 level. When the t statistic was applied, the difference between the two vocabularies for boys was not significant, whereas the difference for girls was significant at the .01 level.

When a Pearson coefficient of correlation was calculated for the two vocabularies the $r = .55$. This is the same value found earlier for cerebral palsied children. A coefficient of this size does not indicate a very strong association.

The correlations with chronological age based on the vocabulary scores of mentally retarded and those based on the scores of cerebral palsied cases show some differences. With the former the correlation of comprehension and chronological age was .24. With the latter it was .80. In the case of the retarded the correlation of expression and chronological age was .01. With the cerebral palsied it was .37.

In relation to mental age the coefficient for the retarded is low. It is $r = .25$, whereas for the cerebral palsied it is .55. The two vocabularies correlate somewhat better with IQ. The correlation with IQ of the vocabulary of comprehension was .60. With expression it was .44.

Cerebral palsied children exceed retarded children on both vocabularies.

The ratio of the vocabulary of comprehension to expression for the mentally retarded was 1.20. The comparable ratio for cerebral palsied children was 1.78.

Three studies were pursued dealing with the proficiency of speech handicapped children to construct sentences. The specific problem was restricted to the number and the length of sentences uttered by these children. The subjects of two of the studies were cerebral palsied children. The third investigated the problem with mentally retarded children.

The sentence for the purpose of this research was defined in the conventional manner as a meaningful word assembly exhibiting a subject and predicate structure with appropriate modifiers. Two aspects of the problem were considered. In one the purpose was to determine the frequency of complete and incomplete or fragmented sentences. The other was to determine the length of sentences used by the children in terms of number of words in both complete and fragmented utterances.

The subjects were sixty-six cerebral palsied children, thirty-three boys and thirty-three girls, who, when tested with familiar pictures, responded with both complete and incomplete utterances. An analysis of variance was run on a 2 by 2 table of the means of complete and incomplete sentences for boys and for girls. It was found that for both boys and girls the means of the complete sentences were larger than the means of the incomplete sentences. The probability value lay at the .025 level. Sex differences were present. The mean of the boys exceeded that of the girls in both the complete and incomplete categories. This is an unusual finding because generally sex differences have not been present throughout the research.

In the second part of this study the number of words used by cerebral palsied subjects in complete and incomplete utterances was determined. The method was to calculate the number of words per sentence per subject. The total number of words was divided by the number of utterances. Thus a child which responded to the set of pictures with five sentences and a total of thirty-five words received a score of 7.0. In this part of the study, sex differences were not present, but for both boys and girls the number of words for complete sentences was significantly greater than for incomplete utterances.

The third study in the series investigated these problems with mentally retarded children. A group of 105 retarded subjects were tested. Of these, sixty—thirty boys and thirty girls—responded with both types of sentences. The reliability of the picture test with the retarded sample was r = .82. With the cerebral palsied group it was .96. The percent of observer reliability was 97.

Using a mixed type of analysis of variance, it was evident that the difference between complete and incomplete utterances of retarded children was inconclusive. The difference between the sexes was not significant. In these two respects the retarded children differed from cerebral palsied children.

The second part of this study concerned the length of the sentence in the speech of these children. Sex difference was significant, and the mean of complete sentences was in excess of the mean of the incomplete sentences.

Mentally retarded and cerebral palsied children then show little difference in the mastery of the sentence.

This section is concerned with the immediate memory spans of mentally retarded children and cerebral palsied children who are mentally retarded. The test used in this study is in three parts, the Wet Fall Test from the Stanford-Binet Intelligence Scale, the Wechsler Intelligence Scale for Children, and the Lost Boy Test constructed for this investigation.

Two hundred eighty-five children from several northwestern states and Canadian Provinces were subjects. An analysis was first made using the composite memory span scores. This was accomplished in two ways. One was according to chronological age, the other according to mental age. All the IQs of this group were below 75. The scores of 523 normal elementary schoolchildren were available for comparative purposes.

According to chronological age levels, there is a significant trend in the means of the scores of the mentally retarded children. In terms of mental age levels there also is a significant trend. However, the mean scores of elementary schoolchildren in grades four to seven exhibit no trend. The means lie on a high plateau. In terms of this test these children apparently have achieved maturity. The average score of this group is about twice the mean score of the retarded group.

A second study of the immediate memory of retarded children was done as a replication of the first study. There were 231 cases from several midwestern states. Additional purposes were to demonstrate that it is feasible to use the verbal and numerical tests as a single test and to learn if the two verbal tests may be used as a single testing instrument. It was found that both questions can be answered affirmatively. Again the sex factor was not apparent.

Comparisons were made between verbal and numerical memory spans at four chronological age levels from 6 to 16 years. None of the mean differences were statistically significant. Similar comparisons were made at four mental age levels. The differences between means at the mental age levels of 2 to 3 years and of 4 to 5 years were significantly in favor of the verbal scores. In subsequent age levels the means were the same.

A third investigation of this variable dealt with other interrelations of the scores of the tests. They were administered to 183 mentally retarded cases, 102 boys and 81 girls. Comparisons were made of boys and girls on each of the three tests, the Wet Fall

Test, the Lost Boy Test and the Digit Span Test. In each the differences were slight and the variances were homogeneous. Further comparisons were run on the means of the three tests based on the scores of boys. The difference between the Wet Fall and Lost Boy tests was slight, but the difference between the Wet Fall and the Digit Span tests was significant at the .001 level. The same was true of the difference between the Lost Boy and Digit Span tests. The same relations were found with girls.

In addition to learning where significant differences among the tests lie, it is of interest to determine the degree of relationships which exists among them. The coefficients of correlation fall within a moderate range. The coefficient for Lost Boy and Digit Span tests is .54. This yields a coefficient of nondetermination of .71. These two tests are therefore fairly unique. The coefficient of correlation for Wet Fall and Digit Span tests was .64.

It may be inferred from the results of the analyses that the two verbal tests may be used as a single testing instrument and that the Digit Span Test adds another dimension to the problem. It was found that mentally retarded cerebral palsied children were superior to mentally retarded children without cerebral palsy.

In a study on manifest anxiety in cerebral palsied children, a scale adapted for use with these children was constructed. Before using the scale, its reliability was determined. Two further problems were investigated: Are cerebral palsied children subject to greater anxiety than non–cerebral-palsied children? Are teachers able to discriminate degrees of anxiety in their pupils?

Seventy-four children were given the test and the means and standard deviations of the odd and even scores were calculated. A t statistic of the difference between the means was determined. The probability value turned out to be .60, evidence of the reliability of the test. Construct validity was provided by the manner in which the items were judged by several speech pathologists.

From the pool of seventy-four children, twenty-seven diagnosed as cerebral palsied were matched on chronological age, mental age and on rated language ability with twenty-seven non–cerebral-palsied children. These included functional cases, stutterers and aphasics. The *t* test indicated that the superiority of the non–cerebral-palsied group which suffered other handicaps was evidenced at the .05 level. This may mean that in their self-evaluation, cerebral palsied children are probably more subject to anxiety than are non–cerebral-palsied children.

One of the aims of this study was to determine if teachers are able to discriminate degrees of anxiety in their pupils. Fifty-eight of the children had been rated by their teachers on a scale of very mild, mild, moderate and severe. An analysis of variance revealed that none of the differences among the means were significant.

In this final part of the recapitulation a number of factors related to the language of speech handicapped children were considered. Interrelationships among the variables studied in this research also were treated.

A composite speech test made up of four tests was administered to 107 cerebral palsied children. It included articulation, sound discrimination, abstraction and vocabulary of comprehension.

The first analysis made with this test concerned sex differences. There was a tendency for boys to exceed girls, but the difference was not significant, p being .55, and the variances were equal. The means of the four tests were found to be quite close to those of previous reports. Thus adding another test to the previous three had little effect.

Spastics and athetoids did equally well on this test. Differences among the means of mildly, moderately and severely involved palsied children did not approach significance. However, according to therapists' ratings of speech and language ability of the children the mean difference of those rated very good and very poor was significant at the .001 level. This study was replicated with 130 children. The replication corroborated the previous results.

The project then was extended in several respects. It included the vocabulary of expression with the four variables. It was further extended to include cerebral palsied children, mentally retarded children, and normal children in elementary school grades. There were 130 cerebral palsied cases, 105 mentally retarded cases, and 318 children in elementary grades.

The schoolchildren were definitely superior to the two handi-capped groups on all five tests. Again on the articulation test the mean of the scores of the retarded was significantly larger than that of the cerebral palsied group. However, for sound discrimi-nation and for abstraction the cerebral palsied children are su-perior. The analysis showed a significant difference between the two groups on both vocabulary of expression and of compre-hension.

Two studies on the intercorrelations of the five tests were done. In one, using 130 cerebral palsied children the coefficients varied from .08 to .67. In a replication with forty subjects they varied from .21 to .67. Generally articulation correlated lowest with the other tests. Sound discrimination in both sets correlated .67 with abstraction. The coefficient of determination then is .45, which suggests that abstraction to a degree involves the process of dis-crimination.

Correlations were run on the scores of the tests and the Wechsler Verbal Scale. Both scales are verbal in nature. Consequently it was considered advisable to learn if the five tests duplicate the WISC. Only one of the five which had a high coefficient with the WISC was the vocabulary of comprehension. The value of r was .94. With articulation, sound discrimination, abstraction and the vo-cabulary of expression the r's were low. They varied from .09 to .49. When the five tests were taken as a unit and were correlated with the WISC Verbal Scale, the coefficient was .50. The coefficient of determination then is .25 and that of nondetermination is .75. This is interpreted to mean that although both are verbal tests, 75% of the variance of the speech variables is independent of the variance of the WISC. These considerations lead to the inference that the variables are related to verbal factors not tapped by the WISC Verbal Scale.

DISCUSSION

In addition to the foregoing summary, certain problems need special consideration.

Attention should be called first to an intriguing anomalous situation. It was found using five different articulation tests, two sound discrimination tests and an abstraction test that the mean differences between right and left hemiplegics was not significant statistically. Moreover the variances of each of eight pairs of samples, with one exception, were homogeneous. In the eight samples there were a total of 242 cases, of which 136 were right and 106 were left hemiplegics. The finding that right and left hemiplegics are alike in their speech performance was unexpected. It is not consistent with the known difference between the anatomy and pathology of the two hemispheres of hemiplegics. Since the speech areas are located mainly in the left hemisphere, it may be expected that its pathology should result in greater speech deficit in right hemiplegics. The results of this investigation, however, do not bear out this expectation. Thus hemiplegics present a special problem.

Quite evidently there is need for better understanding of the interrelationships of neuroanatomy and neuropathology and speech in this type of cerebral palsy. It would be interesting to investigate the possibility or the extent to which in hemiplegics the speech areas are uneffected by pathology in motor areas. The data of the present study throw no light on this problem.

An interesting outcome of the investigation was a tendency exhibited among the consonant profiles toward a fairly close concentration of the percents of articulation errors. This was apparent within the subcategories of the categories of manner, place and voice errors. To illustrate, if the error scores of a child reveal that the difficulty is mainly in the production of palatal sounds it may be profitable for the therapist to work on several of these sounds instead of only one of them at a time. This, of course, is an hypothesis which should be tested by further experimentation. The bearing of manifest anxiety on this problem also should be investigated.

Another interesting finding was that the mean number of word approximations of spastics is about twice their mean number of correct pronunciations. A similar result occurred with athetoids and also with tension athetoids. While correct articulation of sounds by these children was found to be greatly in excess of errors of articulation, errors of pronunciation exceed proper pronunciation of words. Since word approximations are much more frequent in the speech of these children, it is not unreasonable to suggest that the brunt of speech therapy perhaps also should be on pronunciation of whole words rather than on the articulation of single sounds. This likewise is offered as an hypothesis which needs experimental verification.

A significant outcome of these studies is that correct articulation responses for both cerebral palsied and mentally retarded children exceed articulation errors. From the standpoint of speech therapy, this is a hopeful finding.

The order of difficulty of sounds varies between cerebral palsied and mentally retarded children. For other groups, also, it is not the same in the initial, medial and final positions in words. This is also true for educable and trainable mentally retarded.

Another special problem concerns the relative speech abilities of mentally retarded and cerebral palsied children. In regard to articulation two studies were completed, one using a short consonant test, the other the longer Integrated Articulation Test. Comparisons were made at two IQ levels, 25 to 50 and 51 to 80. On the short test the retarded achieved better mean scores than the cerebral palsied children. This was true at both IQ levels. On the long test a similar result was found. It is quite apparent, then, that retarded children have better articulation than cerebral palsied children. In view of the motor deficiency of oral musculature of the cerebral palsied child this result seems reasonable.

The question remains then—Is a similar situation present when communication depends less on motor and more on intellectual or cognitive abilities? This question was investigated with sound discrimination, abstraction, vocabulary, immediate memory span, sentence structure and anxiety testing.

Two studies were done to compare the means of mentally retarded and cerebral palsied children on sound discrimination. In both the mean score of cerebral palsied children significantly exceeded the mean score of the mentally retarded children. A somewhat mixed result was obtained in the abstraction test scores. When the means were based on mental age levels, the differences were not apparent below the 10 to 11 age level. Thereafter the palsied group was superior to the retarded in the ability to perform the cognitive function of abstraction.

The vocabulary of comprehension and expression of cerebral palsied children exceeded that of mentally retarded children. Immediate memory span was better for cerebral palsied children than for mentally retarded children.

Two studies were undertaken to compare mentally retarded and cerebral palsied children in regard to their ability to structure sentences. The mentally retarded and cerebral palsied children were compared in terms of the number and also the length of sentences. In both of them it was found that the two groups were alike both in respect to complete and incomplete sentences. When the study was replicated, similar results were obtained. Thus mentally retarded and cerebral palsied children appear to be alike in their ability to structure sentences.

They were also tested for manifest anxiety. Non–cerebral-palsied children were matched on chronological age, mental age and language ability. The cerebral palsied group made higher scores than the non–cerebral-palsied retarded children. This is interpreted to mean that cerebral palsied children according to their self-evaluation are probably more subject to anxiety than retarded non–cerebral-palsied subjects.

An experiment to determine the effect of anxiety on the other six variables was begun, but before the project could be completed, the research program at the Institute of Logopedics was terminated due to an administrative reorganization. The problem however is critical and needs careful investigation.

Succinctly then, it is indicated in this series of studies that mentally retarded children exceed cerebral palsied children in the functions of articulation. Cerebral palsied children exceed mentally retarded children in sound discrimination, in vocabularies of comprehension and expression, in immediate memory span and manifest anxiety. The two groups perform similarly on tests of number and length of sentences. In the ability to abstract they were alike at younger ages, but after the tenth year the cerebral palsied children were superior. Finally, it may be remarked that the tests used in this research enterprise have had their reliabilities and validities repeatedly established.

This then concludes the examination and evaluation of the seven communication variables, of their components and of their interrelations.

Finally a word needs to be said concerning the possibility of a general theory which will integrate the seven variables considered in this research. It was emphasized that there is substantial independence among them. This view is supported by two different considerations. One is based on statistical evidence, the other on structural linguistic theory. The statistical evidence was presented in the introductory section. There, high coefficients of non-determination afforded information of the weakness of the relations among the variables.

If we turn to linguistics, we find that it does not provide a *general* language theory. Structural linguistics advocates the study of language as an internally organized system. This approach involves an understanding of various levels of linguistic analysis. They are the levels of phonology, morphology and syntax. The sets of rules of analysis for the three levels are not identical. Although the sentence is made up of morphemes and the morphemes are made up of phonemes, each has its own structural rules. Each has its own theory. The rules of grammar do not cover and explain either the morpheme or the phoneme. Heretofore there has been no general or inclusive linguistic theory which successfully integrated the three sets of rules or the several communication variables.

Thus both empirical and theoretical considerations indicate a need for a different mode of integrating the several variables. It was suggested earlier that an effort based on the nature and theory of the construct possibly may resolve the difficulty. A construct is a concept or expression deliberately invented for a special scientific purpose. An instance is the term "articulation." Others are "intelligence," "atom," "motivation," "synapse," "learning," "phoneme," "morpheme," "syntax."

The logic employed in this interpretation holds, as first stated by Margenau (950), that there are two types of concepts or constructs. There are those which are classed as constitutive and those which are categorized as operational. Operational constructs are close to data. They assign meaning by indicating what empirical activities, operations and instructions are needed to identify and measure a variable. The constitutive construct is defined in terms of operationally derived constructs. Communication in this context is interpreted to be an instance of the constitutive type of definition. The seven variables discussed and analyzed in these studies were defined operationally. Factors involved in them were identified and measured, their relationships were processed, and attempts to establish regularities and laws were undertaken. Moreover, the seven variables (and there are others not considered in this investigation) are taken as defining the constitutive construct of communication. A purpose of this book has been to present a body of information processed operationally in order to explicate the construct of communication of speech handicapped children.

PART IX
APPENDIX

A. Description of Subjects

Description of Subjects

Chapter 1

Ninety-six cerebral palsied children were studied. They were in residence in the Iowa Hospital School in Iowa City, the Michael Dowling School in Minneapolis, and the Jamestown North Dakota School. The mean age of the subjects is 8 years, 8 months, and the range is 3 years, 7 months to 15 years, 11 months. In terms of the medical diagnoses, the 96 cases included 41 spastics, 41 athetoids, 1 rigidity, 2 flaccids, 6 ataxic and 5 undetermined. Classified according to extent of involvement, there were 17 mild cases, 35 which were moderate, 40 which were severe cases and 4 cases which were undetermined.

The results of intelligence tests given to the subjects in the three schools are as follows: 19% of the cases which have been given mental tests are mentally defective, half of them fall into the borderline classification, 21% are average and 10% are above average. Thus, about 70% are below average. The majority of the subjects were tested with Form L of the Stanford-Binet Scale; a few were given the Wechsler Intelligence Scale for Children.

Chapter 6

In this study data were secured on 226 children with cerebral palsy from the states of Tennessee, South Carolina, Georgia, Florida, Alabama, Louisiana and Iowa. In terms of the medical diagnosis they fell into the following categories:

Spastic	120
Athetoid	70
Ataxic	18
Rigid	2
Tremor	3
Mixed	4
Undetermined	9

The classification according to extent of involvement was

Quadriplegic	153
Paraplegic	23
Hemiplegic	27
Triplegic	8
Diplegic	1
Monoplegic	4
Undetermined	10

The distribution according to the degree of involvement was

Mild	56
Moderate	82
Severe	88

The chronological age range was 3½ to 19 years, the mean age being 9½ years. The IQs were distributed into five groups:

	%	F
Below 40	10	6
41–70	49	31
71–90	56	35
91–110	41	26
111+	4	2
Undetermined	66	—

Chapter 9

There were 103 children with cerebral palsy who were subjects in this investigation. They were from the states of Kansas, Oklahoma, Texas, New Mexico, Arizona and California. They ranged in chronological age from 3 to 16 years with a mean of 9 years, 6 months. The mean mental age was 7 years, 2 months, with a range of 3 to 14 years.

Classified according to the medical diagnosis there were

Spastic	61
Athetoid	14
Tension Athetoid	5
Rigid	1
Flaccid	1
Tremor	1
Ataxic	8
Mixed	6
Undetermined	6

The distribution according to the extent of involvement was

Quadriplegic	58
Paraplegic	13
Hemiplegic	18
Triplegic	3

Monoplegic	4
Undetermined	6

The grouping according to degree of involvement was

Mild	30
Moderate	35
Severe	31
Undetermined	6

The distribution according to general speech and language ratings was

Good	31
Medium	36
Poor	24
Not rated	11

The IQs of these children were distributed in four categories:

	F	$\%$
41–70	18	26
71–90	31	46
91–110	12	18
111+	7	10
Undetermined	35	—

Chapter 12

The subjects were from the states of Maine, Vermont, New Hampshire, Massachusetts, Connecticut, Florida, Alabama, Mississippi, Louisiana, Texas and Arkansas. One hundred sixty children with cerebral palsy were subjects in the experiment. They ranged in chronological age from 2 to 17 years with a mean of 8 years, 10 months. The mean mental age was 6 years with a range of 2 years, 6 months, to 13 years, 10 months.

Classified according to the medical diagnosis there were

Spastic	96
Athetoid	27
Tension Athetoid	7
Rigid	1
Flaccid	1
Ataxic	5
Mixed	6
Undetermined	17

The distribution according to extent of involvement was

Quadriplegic	82
Paraplegic	32
Hemiplegic, Right	15
Hemiplegic, Left	15
Triplegic	4

Undetermined 11

The grouping according to degree of involvement was

Mild	35
Moderate	49
Severe	68
Undetermined	8

The IQ's of the children were distributed in five categories. There were 114 children to whom mental tests were administered.

	F	%
1–40	5	4.4
41–70	39	34.2
71–90	42	36.8
91–110	23	20.2
111+	5	4.4
Undetermined	46	—

About 75% of these cerebral palsied children had IQs below 90. It was reported in a previous section that about 72% had IQs below 90.

Chapter 14

The 136 cerebral palsied children fell into the following medical categories:

Spastic	81
Athetoid	20
Tension Athetoid	4
Ataxic	2
Rigid	2
Mixed	6
Undetermined	14

The classification according to extent of involvement is

Quadriplegic	62
Paraplegic	24
Hemiplegic	21
Triplegic	2
Undetermined	20

The categories according to degree of involvement are

Mild	33
Moderate	37
Severe	54
Undetermined	5

Chapter 19

The children who were subjects in part one were from the states of Arkansas, Florida, Iowa, Kansas, Minnesota and Missouri.

There was a total of 134 subjects with a chronological age range of 3 to 16 years. The mean age was 9.3 years. The mean mental age was 5.4 years with a range of 2 to 9 years.

The distribution according to the medical diagnosis was as follows:

Spastic	44
Athetoid	20
Tension Athetoid	3
Rigid	3
Ataxic	7
Mixed	5
Undetermined	32*

The grouping according to the degree of involvement was

Mild	35
Moderate	22
Severe	26
Undetermined	31

Speech therapists rated 76 of the children on a three-point scale as good, medium and poor on general language ability and speech intelligibility. The distribution follows:

Good	29
Medium	17
Poor	40

Chapter 20

The children were from the states of Arkansas, Florida, Iowa, Kansas, Minnesota, Missouri, New Mexico, North Carolina, North Dakota, Oklahoma, South Dakota and Wisconsin. The mean chronological age was 9.1 years with a range of 3 to 16 years. The mean mental age was 5.2 years, the range being 1.5 to 9 years. The mean IQ was 78.4 with a range extending from 17 to 134.

According to the medical diagnosis there were

Spastic	84
Athetoid	23
Tension Athetoid	6
Rigid	2
Ataxic	7
Mixed	8
Undetermined	36
Total	166

*The large number of undeterminates in this study is due to the incompleteness of records in the original files at various centers.

Classified according to extent of involvement there were

Quadriplegic	82
Paraplegic	16
Hemiplegic	29
Triplegic	5
Undetermined	34

The grouping according to degree of involvement was

Mild	53
Moderate	35
Severe	52
Undetermined	26

The IQs of these children were distributed in five categories. There were 105 children to whom mental tests were administered.

	F	%
1 – 40	3	2
41 – 70	31	30
71 – 90	39	37
91 – 110	28	27
111 +	4	4
Undetermined	61	—

About 70% of these cerebral palsied children had IQs below 90 and about 30% were below 70.

Chapter 24

The classification of the cerebral palsied children in sample 1 according to the medical diagnosis has been reported elsewhere. The classification of the combined samples is as follows:

	F	%
Spastic	147	55.0
Athetoid	59	22.0
Tension Athetoid	7	3.0
Ataxic	15	6.0
Flaccid	2	0.5
Rigid	3	1.0
Tremor	1	0.5
Mixed	21	8.0
Undetermined	10	4.0
	265	100.0

The distribution of the combined samples according to extent of involvement is

	F	%
Quadriplegic	154	58
Paraplegic	43	16
Hemiplegic	36	14

Triplegic	6	2
Undetermined	26	10
	265	100

Grouping according to degree of involvement

	F	%
Mild	93	35
Moderate	85	32
Severe	72	27
Undetermined	15	6
	265	100

Grouped according to general speech and language ability as rated by the speech therapist

	F	%
Very Good	34	13
Good	66	25
Medium	64	24
Poor	48	18
Very Poor	41	15
Undetermined	12	5
	265	100

The mental status of the children is indicated by the following IQ categories:

	F	%
1 – 40	19	11
41 – 70	52	29
71 – 90	65	38
91 – 110	32	19
111 – plus	6	3
Undetermined	91	—

There were 178 of the cerebral palsied children in the two samples to whom mental tests had been administered. Of these only 22% were normal or above normal and 11% were below IQ 40. The other 78% of the children had IQs below 90. Thus a majority of the children, in addition to being afflicted with cerebral palsy, were mentally retarded.

Chapter 28

One hundred and five subjects were utilized in this investigation. They were divided into the following groups:

A. Educable Mentally Retarded

This group was composed of 41 retarded children. There were

28 boys and 13 girls. Their IQs ranged from 46 to 88 with a mean of 66.80. The IQs were all determined by the Stanford-Binet, Form L. The chronological ages ranged from 7 years, 1 month, to 12 years, 6 months. The mean age was 9 years, 9 months. This group was part of a group of 45 educable retarded children enrolled in three classes organized for extensive study by the State University of Iowa, the Iowa State Department of Public Instruction, and the U.S. Office of Health, Education and Welfare. As a part of this broader study, the children had been given complete physical examinations as well as hearing tests. No subjects were used who were suspected of having brain damage or hearing losses. Four subjects from the larger group were not included for these reasons. One boy was cerebral palsied, one girl had a repaired cleft palate and two others transferred out of the school system before completion of this study. This was a relatively homogeneous sample of educable mentally retarded, non–brain-damaged schoolchildren.

B. Matched Control Group of Normal Children

A matched group of 41 normal children was selected to serve as controls. They were matched within age groups with the educable retarded children. The control group was selected to meet the following specifications:

1. Otis Quick Scoring Mental Ability IQs were to be between 90 to 110. (One boy was selected whose IQ was 88. This was made necessary by the limited number of boys who met all requirements.)
2. The subjects were to fall within the same chronological age levels as were in the sample of retarded children.
3. Each subject's socioeconomic rating was to be in the same range of ratings as in the educable retarded sample.

Cumulative records of children in Cedar Rapids were studied and a sample obtained which met the above specifications. From these records a small sample was randomly chosen until each age level of the retarded had an equivalent number of matched normal subjects.

Matching on the basis of socioeconomic ratings was especially useful in this study on articulation for Templin (1957) found significant differences between the ability of upper-class and lower-class children to articulate speech sounds. Since this variable has been controlled, differences between the two groups cannot be attributed to social class differences.

C. *Trainable Mentally Retarded*

This sample was drawn from two locations: the Vineland Training School, Vineland, New Jersey, and a private school for retarded children at Nashua, New Hampshire. The group was composed of 23 children. The chronological ages ranged from 7 to 14 years with a mean of 10 years, 5 months. Their IQs ranged from 25 to 47 with a mean IQ of 38.

Chapter 30

Data were collected on 333 children with cerebral palsy from New England and southern states. Classified according to the medical diagnosis they fall into the following categories:

Spastic	187
Athetoid	63
Tension Athetoid	14
Ataxic	12
Rigid	4
Flaccid	2
Tremor	0
Mixed	18
Undetermined	33

The distribution according to extent of involvement is

Quadriplegic	189
Paraplegic	48
Hemiplegic	53
Triplegic	6
Undetermined	37

The following categories are according to degree of involvement:

Mild	79
Moderate	124
Severe	114
Undetermined	16

Chapter 33

The subjects were handicapped children receiving therapy in

the Institute. The mean age was 11 years, 1 month, and the range was from 6 years to 17 years, 7 months. Most of them were residents in the Institute. There were 95 males and 44 females. They were children with a variety of speech problems as presented in the following tabulation.

	F	%
Normal	13	9
Borderline	16	12
Educable	31	22
Trainable	13	9
Cerebral Palsied	45	33
Miscellaneous	21	15
	139	100

The tabulation indicates that 9% are mentally normal and 43% are below normal. The cerebral palsied and miscellaneous group comprise the remaining 48%. Among the miscellaneous group about half were functional cases, the others were stutterers, a few had cleft palates, and there were single cases of other diagnoses. Forty-five or about half of the entire sample were cerebral palsied children. Thus the sample included a wide variety of problems.

The speech and language ability of the children were rated by the therapist as follows:

	F	%
Very Good	21	15
Good	54	39
Medium	43	31
Poor	20	14
Very Poor	1	1
	139	100

Chapter 34

Form A was administered to 153 children with cerebral palsy from 6 through 16 years of age with a mean chronological age of 10.3 years. The mean mental age was 6.5 years, the range was 2.8 to 17.0 years. They were from speech centers, public schools and hospitals in eleven states.

According to the medical diagnosis the subjects are grouped as follows:

	F	%
Spastic	95	62

Athetoid	30	19
Tension Athetoid	4	2
Ataxic	7	4
Rigid	4	2
Mixed	11	7
Undetermined	2	1

According to extent of involvement the following is the distribution:

	F	%
Quadriplegic	78	51
Paraplegic	34	22
Hemiplegic	34	20
Triplegic	2	1
Undetermined	10	6

The distribution in terms of degree of involvement is

	F	%
Mild	39	25
Moderate	56	37
Severe	55	36
Undetermined	3	2

Grouped according to general speech and language ability as rated by the speech therapist:

	F	%
Very Good	27	18
Good	44	29
Medium	25	16
Poor	29	19
Very Poor	22	14
Undetermined	6	4

Distribution according to IQ categories:

	F	%
1 – 40	3	2
41 – 70	47	31
71 – 90	43	28
91 – 110	26	17
111 +	7	4
Undetermined*	27	18

*The fact that in these several distributions an "undetermined" category is included means that in subsequent analysis different Ns will be used.

Chapter 35

Form B was administered to 260 cerebral palsied children in two geographical regions. One included the states of Colorado, Idaho, Montana, Oregon, Utah and Washington; the other Iowa,

Minnesota, North Dakota, Nebraska and South Dakota. The age range was from 6 to 17 years with a mean chronological age of 10.9 years. The mean mental age was 6.8 years and the range was 1.7 to 15.1 years.

According to the medical diagnosis the distribution of the subjects was as follows:

	F	%
Spastic	136	52.0
Athetoid	51	20.0
Tension Athetoid	17	7.0
Ataxic	11	4.0
Rigid	1	0.5
Flaccid	1	0.5
Mixed	32	12.0
Undetermined	11	4.0

According to extent of involvement the subjects are grouped as follows:

	F	%
Quadriplegic	168	65
Paraplegic	28	11
Hemiplegic	35	13
Triplegic	6	2
Undetermined	23	9

The distribution in terms of degree of involvement is

	F	%
Mild	48	19
Moderate	83	32
Severe	92	35
Undetermined	37	14

Ratings by the speech therapist of general speech and language ability are

	F	%
Very Good	34	13
Good	73	28
Medium	55	21
Poor	49	19
Very Poor	39	15
Undetermined	10	4

Distribution according to IQ categories is

	F	%
1 – 40	2	1
41 – 70	52	20
71 – 90	100	39
91 – 110	63	24
111 +	11	4

Undetermined*   32   12

---

*Nonbrain injured includes familial or "garden-variety" and subcultural types of defectives. These diagnoses, including the brain injured were identified from medical records. The epileptic group was also mentally retarded.

Chapter 36

In this sample a total of 357 mentally retarded children from 6 to 17 years old were examined with Form A of a Sound Discrimination Test originally designed for use with cerebral palsied children. The subjects were from the following states: Arkansas, California, Colorado, Connecticut, Kansas, Missouri and West Virginia. In order to respond to the items of the test the child had to be able to distinguish between the sound of the word "same" and "different." Of the 357 cases, 166 were able to do this. The following analyses were done on the 166 cases. A separate analysis is being made of the remaining cases.

It should be born in mind that there is no generally accepted classification of types of mental retardation. According to a medical classification, the subjects of this study are arbitrarily grouped as follows:

	F	%
Nonbrain Injured*	77	46
Brain Injured*	31	18
Mongol	4	3
Cretin	1	1
Epileptic*	15	9
Hydrocephalic	2	1
Microcephalic	1	1
Undetermined	35	21
	166	100
	F	%
Educables	119	76
Trainables	37	24
	156	100

---

*Not all the children were given mental tests.

Chapter 39

The frequency and percent of frequency of the types of 142

subjects with cerebral palsy in the final sample are tabulated in the following:

	F	%
Spastic	91	64
Athetoid	34	24
Ataxic	4	3
Tremor	1	1
Mixed	10	7
Undetermined	2	1
	142	100

The distribution according to extent of involvement is

	F	%
Quadriplegic	83	58
Paraplegic	21	15
Hemiplegic	24	17
Triplegic	3	2
Diplegic	3	2
Undetermined	8	6
	142	100

Grouping according to degree of involvement is

	F	%
Mild	45	32
Moderate	47	33
Severe	48	34
Undetermined	2	1
	142	100

Grouping according to general speech and language ability

	F	%
Very Good	17	12
Good	39	28
Medium	36	25
Poor	29	20
Very Poor	21	15
	142	100

Seventy-two of the 142 cerebral palsied children were given the Peabody Picture Test. The distribution of their IQs is indicated by the following IQ categories:

	F	%
1 – 40	4	5
41 – 70	15	21
71 – 90	29	40
91 – 100	17	24
111 – plus	7	10
	72	100

Sixty-eight of the children were given the Similarities Test of the Weschsler Intelligence Scale for Children. The distribution according to the categories of scores is given in the following:

	F	%
0 – 1	5	7
1 – 4	20	30
5 – 8	17	25
9 – 12	23	35
13 – 18	3	3
	68	100

Chapter 40

Form X of the test was given to 109 mentally retarded children in several northwestern states and in the state of Hawaii who were attending public schools and state hospitals for retarded children. The performance of 97 of them was suitable for use in this study. The remaining twelve children did not respond to the testing situation. The mean chronological age of the children was 12 years, 5 months, and the range was 6 to 17 years. Since Abstraction Test utilizes auditory input, the adequacy of hearing of the subjects was determined by an audiometer or by a spondee test. The criterion was ability to hear in a conversational setting.

The diagnoses of mental retardation were obtained from medical records at the various facilities where the data were collected. Accordingly the following medical classification was based on their records.

	F	%
Nonbrain Injury	36	37
Brain Injury	31	32
Hydrocephaly	1	1
Microcephaly	1	1
Epilepsy	4	4
Undetermined	24	25
	97	100

Chapter 42

Ninety-one cerebral palsied children, 44 boys and 47 girls, were subjects in this experiment. The chronological age range was 5 to 17 years, 5 months, the mean being 10 years, 6 months. The mental range was from 2 years, 3 months, to 11 years, 4 months.

The mean mental age was 9 years, 7 months. The subjects were from the provinces of Manitoba and Ontario, Canada.

The frequency and percent of frequency of the types of cerebral palsy are given in the following tabulation:

	F	%
Spastic	65	71
Athetoid	16	17
Ataxic	6	7
Mixed	4	5
	91	100

The distribution according to extent of involvement is

	F	%
Quadriplegics	56	61
Hemiplegic	12	13
Paraplegic	17	19
Triplegic	4	5
Monoplegic	2	2
	91	100

Grouping according to degree of involvement is

	F	%
Mild	23	25
Moderate	39	43
Severe	27	30
Undetermined	2	2
	91	100

Distribution according to general speech and language ability as rated by therapists:

	F	%
Very Good	6	7
Good	24	26
Medium	20	22
Poor	21	23
Very Poor	4	4
Undetermined	16	18
	91	100

Chapter 52

The children were from the states of Arizona, California, Kansas, Oklahoma, New Mexico and Texas. They ranged in age from 5 years, 9 months, to 17 years, 6 months, the mean being 10 years, 9 months. Children with hearing losses were excluded from the sample. The diagnoses of cerebral palsy were taken from the medical records found in the children's cumulative folders. The following classification of the types of cerebral palsy was based on these records.

	F	%
Spastics	73	68
Athetoids	16	15
Mixed	13	12
Ataxics	3	3
Rigidites	2	2
	107	100

The distribution according to the extent of involvement is

	F	%
Quadriplegic	72	67
Hemiplegic	16	15
Paraplegic	10	9
Monoplegic	6	6
Undetermined	3	3
	107	100

The distribution according to degree of involvement is

	F	%
Mild	33	31
Moderate	30	28
Severe	24	22
Undetermined	20	19
	107	100

The distribution according to general speech and language as rated by speech therapists is

	F	%
Very Good	22	20
Good	33	31
Medium	30	28
Poor	15	14
Very Poor	3	3
Undetermined	4	4
	107	100

Chapter 55

Five speech tests were administered to 130 cerebral palsied children from three western provinces of Canada and three northwestern states. They ranged in age from 6 years, 4 months, to 16 years, 9 months. The mean age was 10 years, 11 months. The classification of cerebral palsy were according to type, extent of involvement, degree of involvement and speech therapists' ratings as found in the medical records of the childrens' folders.

The frequency and percent of frequency of the types of cerebral palsy are given in the following tabulation:

	F	%
Spastics	72	55
Athetoids	25	19
Tension Athetoid	4	3
Rigid	3	3
Ataxic	4	3
Mixed	14	11
Undetermined	8	6
	130	100

The distribution according to extent of involvement is

	F	%
Quadriplegic	72	55
Paraplegic	25	19
Right Hemiplegic	11	9
Left Hemiplegic	5	4
Triplegic	2	1
Monoplegic	2	1
Undetermined	13	11
	130	100

Grouping according to degree of involvement is

	F	%
Mild	29	22
Moderate	38	29
Severe	35	27
Undetermined	28	22
	130	100

Distribution according to therapists' ratings is

	F	%
Very Good	14	11
Good	40	31
Medium	29	22
Poor	19	15
Very Poor	6	4
Undetermined	22	17
	130	100

The other samples of children, one of forty cerebral palsied subjects, the other of eighty speech handicapped children were comparable to the 130 children in ranges of chronological age. Among the sample of eighty subjects, twenty-eight were cerebral palsied and fifty-two were aphasic.

B. Charts

CHART 1

Part Test A. Consonants

Items		Alternates
1. ball	b–	boy
2. bed	–d	bird
3. rabbit	–b–	baby
4. tub	–b	club
5. cup	–p	soup
6. ice cream	–m	comb
7. milk	m–	man
8. pig	p–	pie
9. hat	–t	coat
10. mama	–m–	umbrella
11. kitten	–t–	butter
12. dog	d–	duck
13. candy	–d–	candle
14. table	t–	tree
15. apple	–p–	puppy

CHART 2

Part Test B. Consonants

Items		Alternatives	
1. dog	–g	pig	
2. cat	k–	cow	
3. bathe	–ð	breathe	
4. foot	f–	face	
			f
5. gun	g–	girl	
			v
6. sugar	–g–	cigar	ð
7. basket	–k–	biscuit	
8. very	v–	vase	ɵ
			g
9. knife	–f	wife	
			k
10. seven	–v–	clover	
11. that	ð–	them	
12. thin	ɵ–	thumb	
13. feather	–ð–	mother	
14. Kathy	–ɵ–	bathtub	
15. sofa	–f–	rifle	
16. stove	–v	serve	
17. book	–k	coke	
18. path	–ɵ	teeth	

339

CHART 3

Part Test B. Consonants

1.	car	–r		s
2.	leg	l–		z
3.	dish	–ʃ		ʃ
4.	so	s–		ʒ
5.	red	r–		r
6.	carry	–r–		l
7.	hello	–l–		
8.	zoo	z–		
9.	us	–s		
10.	easy	–z–		
11.	she	ʃ–		
12.	fishes	–ʃ–		
13.	usual	–ʒ–		
14.	lesson	–s–		
15.	has	–z		
16.	ball	–l		
17.	garage	–ʒ		

CHART 4

Vowel Test

1.	bean –i–	i	11.	did –I–	
2.	Ed ɛ	I	12.	cut –ʌ–	
3.	cook –u–	ɛ	13.	oak o–	
4.	eat i–	æ	14.	at æ–	
5.	can æ	ʌ	15.	noon –u–	
6.	bed –ɛ–	ɝ	16.	ball –ɔ–	
7.	up ʌ–	ɑ	17.	doll –ɑ–	
8.	all ɔ–	ɔ	18.	on ɑ–	
9.	coke –o–	o	19.	ooze u–	
10.	in I–	U	20.	bird ɝ	
		u			

CHART 5

Vowels in Single and Two Syllable Words

1.	–i–	bean	i	13.	–i–	beneath
2.	–I–	did	I	14.	–I–	begin
3.	–e–	bake	e	15.	–e–	behave
4.	–ɛ–	bed	ɛ	16.	–ɛ–	again
5.	–æ–	can	æ	17.	–æ–	canal
6.	–ʌ–	cut	ʌ	18.	–ʌ–	enough
7.	–ɝ–	bird	ɝ	19.	ɝ	deserve
8.	–a–	doll	ɑ	20.	–ɑ–	garage
9.	–ɔ–	ball	ɔ	21.	–ɔ–	belong
10.	–o–	coke	o	22.	–o–	suppose
11.	–U–	cook	U	23.	–U–	mistook
12.	–u–	moon	u	24.	–u–	balloon

CHART 6

Vowell Test, Form I

1.	–i–	bean	i	11.	–I–	did
2.	ɛ–	Ed	I	12.	–ʌ–	cut
3.	–u–	cook	e	13.	–O–	oak
4.	i–	eat	ɛ	14.	–æ–	at
5.	–æ–	can	æ	15.	–u–	moon
6.	–ɛ–	bed	ʌ	16.	–ɔ–	ball
7.	ʌ–	up	ɝ	17.	–ɑ–	doll
8.	ɔ–	all	ɑ	18.	ɑ–	on
9.	–O–	coke	O	19.	u–	ooze
10.	I–	in	U	20.	ɝ	bird
			u			
			ɔ			

CHART 7

Vowel Test, Form II

1.	ɛ–	elm	i	11.	–ɑ–	bomb
2.	u–	oodles	I	12.	–u–	spoon
3.	I–	it	e	13.	ʌ–	under
4.	–U–	book	ɛ	14.	O–	old
5.	–ɛ–	pet	æ	15.	ɑ–	olive
6.	–i–	bead	ʌ	16.	i–	eel
7.	æ–	add	ɝ	17.	–O–	note
8.	–ʌ–	gun	ɑ	18.	–æ–	cat
9.	ɔ–	auto	ɔ	19.	–ɑ–	tall
10.	–I–	tin	O	20.	–ɝ–	hurt
			U			
			u			

CHART 8

Diphthongs

1.	boy	–ɔI	oU	8.	ate	eI–
2.	pie	–aI	aU	9.	ride	–aI–
3.	loud	–aU	eI	10.	eye	aI–
4.	hay	–eI	aI	11.	boat	–oU–
5.	tail	–eI	ɔI	12.	out	aU–
6.	noise	–ɔI		13.	toe	–oU
7.	cow	–aU–		14.	oat	oU–

CHART 9

Score Sheet According to Place, Manner and Voicing

(Refer to page 122 for Chart 9.)

CHART 10
Ten Most Difficult Consonants

1.	–z	has	s	16.	–ʃ–	fishes
2.	r–	red	z	17.	dʒ	jack
3.	–s	us	dʒ	18.	–t	hat
4.	–ө–	Kathy	tʃ	19.	–dʒ	age
5.	s–	so	ө	20.	–tʃ	teacher
6.	z–	zoo	ʃ	21.	–ʃ	dish
7.	ʃ–	she	ð	22.	–dʒ–	pigeon
8.	–t–	kitten	r	23.	–i–	hello
9.	–tʃ	much	t	24.	tʃ–	chair
10.	t–	table	l	25.	–z–	easy
11.	ө–	thin		26.	–ө	path
12.	–r	car		27.	–ð	bathe
13.	–ð–	feather		28.	–s–	lesson
14.	–r–	carry		29.	l–	leg
15.	–ð–	that		30.	–l	ball

CHART 11
Test of Ten Consonants

1.	s–	soap		16.	dʒ–	jam
2.	z–	zone	s	17.	–ʃ	wish
3.	–s	hiss	z	18.	–t	bat
4.	–ө–	nothing	dʒ	19.	–dʒ–	magic
5.	–s–	essay	tʃ	20.	–t–	bitten
6.	t–	tell	ө	21.	–ʃ–	ashes
7.	–z	his	ʃ	22.	ð–	than
8.	–tʃ	rich	ð	23.	–dʒ	cage
9.	–ө	both	r	24.	–ʃ	fall
10.	–z–	breezy	t	25.	ʃ–	sheep
11.	–ð	breathe	l	26.	–ð–	father
12.	ө–	thick		27.	ʃ–	left
13.	r–	rent		28.	tʃ–	chick
14.	–ʃ–	yellow		29.	–r	far
15.	–r–	story		30.	–tʃ–	butcher

CHART 12
Form A. Individual Record Sheet

A Sound Discrimination Test for Use with Children with Cerebral Palsy

Name _____ Institution _____ Date_____

Instruction: I am going to say two words. Sometimes the words will be the same. Then you say "same." Sometimes parts of the words will be the same but other parts will be different. Then you say "different." Let's try some words. Practice items: ma-pa, boy-toy, tune-loon, moon-moon, for-door, leave-leash.

Items	Correct	Error	No Response
1. tin-thin			
2. late-date			
3. pig-big			
4. (gun-gun)			
5. test-text			

6.	bud-bug		
7.	chip-ship		
8.	habitat-habitant		
9.	sop-ship		
10.	conical-comical		
11.	(hoe-hoe)		
12.	beats-beads		
13.	cytology-psychology		
14.	class-clasp		
15.	mush-much		
16.	patriarch-matriarch		
17.	(peach-peach)		
18.	wear-where		
19.	biscuit-brisket		
20.	foal-stole		
21.	pass-path		
22.	convergent-conversant		
23.	falls-false		
24.	(at-at)		
25.	refracted-retracted		
26.	coke-cope		
27.	carrion-Marion		
28.	(far-far)		
29.	frisking-whisking		
30.	thigh-sigh		

Attention Good   Repetition

Yes _____ No_____   Yes _____ No_____

Do not include items in parentheses in the total score.

Totals: Correct _____ Error _____ No Response _____

Administered by _____ Tabulated by _____

CHART 13

Form B. Individual Sheet

A Sound Discrimination Test for Use with Children with Cerebral Palsy

Name _____ Institution _____ Date_____

Instruction: I am going to say two words. Sometimes the words will be the same. Then you say "same." Sometimes parts of the words will be the same but other parts will be different. Then you say "different." Let's try some words. Practice items: *ma-pa, boy-toy, tune-loon, moon-moon, for-door, leave-leash.*

Items	*Correct*	*Error*	*No Response*
1. leech-leash			
2. church-birch			
3. wench-wrench			
4. antecedent-antecedence			
5. (late-late)			
6. defection-deflection			
7. retraction-detraction			
8. hydrolyte-hydrolize			
9. splashing-flashing			
10. (unearth-unearch)			
11. tub-tug			

12. slough*s*-slui*ce*
13. impelle*nt*-impelle*r*
14. hur*t*ing-her*d*ing
15. *d*enominate-*r*enominate
16. *ch*oke-*j*oke
17. (*b*room-*b*room)
18. *f*resh-*f*lesh
19. wrea*th*-wrea*the*
20. grie*v*e-grie*f*
21. ma*tt*er-ma*dd*er
22. (*ath*lete-*ath*lete)
23. boo*t*-booe*d*
24. mo*bb*ing-mo*pp*ing
25. hydrochlori*c*-hydrochlori*d*
26. key*ed*-kee*n*
27. (poe*m*-poe*m*)
28. rheo*scope*-rheo*trope*
29. oscillogra*ph*-oscillogra*m*
30. *p*receding-*r*eceding

Attention Good   Repetition
  Yes _____ No_____   Yes _____ No_____
Do not include items in parentheses in the total score.
Totals: Correct _____ Error _____ No Response _____
Administered by _____ Tabulated by _____

CHART 14

Form X. A Test of Abstraction for Use with Cerebral Palsied Children

Name........................ Center............................. Sex   M F
          Last   First
                        Totals   Year   Month   Day
          Correct: ......   Date: ....
          Error: ......   Born: ....
          No Response: ......   Age: ....

Administered by........................Tabulated by......................

General Instructions to the Examiner

The examiner on giving instructions to the child is requested to repeat them without deviation. Lettered items are for practice and may be repeated until the examiner is certain that the child understands. Numbered items may be repeated once if the child does not hear or is not attending, but not if the initial response is in error. Circle the answer given by the child.

Instructions to the Child

"I am going to say some sentences. In each sentence you will hear four words such as: dog, cat, pencil and pony. Dog, cat and pony are animals. They belong together, but pencil is not an animal so it does not belong with the animals. Now I am going to say some more sentences, and I want you to tell me which word does not belong."

a. Which word does not belong: hat, **boat,** shoes, coat?
b. Which does not belong: car, train, ship, **mountain**?

Note

In case of failure on practice item a, the examiner will need to explain, "Hat, shoes, and coat are articles of clothing and go together; but one does not wear a boat. It does not belong with the other items."

1. Which does not belong: worm, **stick**, fish, bird?
2. Which does not belong: man, boy, baby, **kitty?**
3. Which does not belong: chair, **truck,** rug, table?

Instructions to the Child

"Now these will be a little different."
c. A horse is: an automobile, **an animal**, a feather, a kite.
d. A banana is: red, hard, sharp, **yellow.**
"Now let's go on."

4. A baseball is: **round,** sour, hot, mushy.
5. Light is: what you hear, what you feel, **what you see,** what you eat.
6. A pony is: a small wagon, **a small horse,** a small tiger, a small car.
7. The sky is **blue,** green, narrow, greasy.
8. A grape is: **round,** hard, bitter, woody.
9. Which is longer than a month: hour, week, **year,** day?
10. Which is heavier than a dog: a mouse, **a horse,** an ant, a canary?
11. Which is longest: an inch, a foot, **a mile,** a yard?
12. What month does Christmas come in: September, May, January, **December.**
13. What number is more than seven: 2, 6, **9,** 4?
14. What number is more than eleven: 10, 9, **12,** 7?
15. Which word goes with automobile: sky, post, **wheel,** horse?
16. Which word tells about the doctor: floor, **medicine,** snow, rain?
17. Which word tells about light: itch, beans, **sun,** dress?
18. Which word tells about the sky: garden, **star,** street, tree?
19. Which tells about sharp: balloon, **knife,** stone, book?
20. Which word tells about the sun: rain, **light,** cold, dark?
21. A circle is made of: **one line,** five lines, three lines, four lines.

Instructions to the Child

"I am going to say four words. Two of the words will be more alike than the other two."
e. Which are more alike: **dog and cat** or cat and table?

Note

In case of error on the example, the examiner will need to explain "Dog and cat are both animals, they are alike; but cat and table are not alike at all." If the child responds with one of the pair and not the other, it is an error.

22. Which are more alike: **Heel and toe** or chair and house?
23. Which are more alike: river and sky or **book and newspaper?**
24. Which are more alike: **snow and ice** or flag and tree?
25. Which are more alike: horse and flower or **milk and water?**

Attention Good   **Repetition**
    Yes . . . . . . No . . . . . .   Yes . . . . . . No . . . . . .

CHART 15

The Lost Boy Test

Instructions: Here is a story about a lost boy. Listen carefully because when I have finished reading it, I want you to tell it. Here is the story: "The Lost Boy."

If a boy is lost. He should stand quietly and not run. First he must look for a policeman or a friendly man or woman. Then he must tell that person he does not know where he is, and give his name and street number if he can remember it. The person will do everything to find the boy's parents.

The following questions are presented to the subject after the story has been read:

1. What is the name of this story?
2. What should a lost boy do?

3. What should he look for?
4. What must he tell?
5. What must he remember?
6. What will happen?

CHART 16

A Manifest Anxiety Scale for Use With Cerebral Palsied Children

Instructions: Make a check mark before the "yes" answers.

1. Are you afraid in the dark?
2. Are you afraid of falling?
   (Do you ever get mad?)
3. Does it bother you because you can't play games with other children?
4. Does it bother you to take this test?
5. Are you ever worried about yourself?
   (Are you always good?)
6. Do you worry about your parents?
   (Are you a boy?)
7. Are you ever troubled because its hard for you to talk?
8. Are you nervous in crowded streets?
9. Does it bother you to talk to grown-up people?
10. Do you worry when you are sick?
11. Do you have to go to the toilet more than most people?
12. Does it bother you when you spill your food?
13. Are you shy or afraid of strangers?
    (Are you a horse?)
14. Do you dislike going to class?
15. Are you scared when a bigger boy (or girl) hits you?
16. Do you worry when you go to bed at night?
    (Do you like candy?)
17. Do you often get lonesome?
    (Do you like Christmas?)
18. Do you have trouble swallowing?
19. Do you have trouble getting your breath?
    (Do you eat stones?)
20. Do you get headaches?
    (What kind of things bother you?)

Foils are included in order to determine if the child is perseverating.

Number of "yes" responses _____

CHART 17

Test Items for Control of Speech Mechanisms

	Number of times in 1 minute
A. **Tongue**	
1. Move tip below lower lip	. . . .
2. Move tip above upper lip	. . . .
3. Move tip from corner to corner of mouth	. . . .
4. Move tip against lower teeth	

5. Move tip against upper teeth   . . . .

B. Lips

    1. Extend corners of lips backward from forward
       rounded position (teeth together)   . . . .
    2. Open and close lips (teeth together)   . . . .

C. Mandible

    1. Open and close mouth (jaw and lips move together)   . . . .

D. Respiration

    1. Sustain even phonation of the sound a for 10 seconds   . . . .
    2. Sustain even silent exhilation for 10 seconds   . . . .

C. Record Forms

INDIVIDUAL RECORD SHEET
Cerebral Palsy
Part Test A. Consonants

Name_____ Institution_____ Date_____

		Correct	Substitution	Omitted	Distorted	No Response	Neutral*
1. ball	b–						
2. bed	–d						
3. rabbit	–b–						
4. tub	–b						
5. cup	–p						
6. home	–m						
7. milk	m–						
8. pig	p–						
9. hat	–t						
10. mama	–m–						
11. kitten	–t–						
12. dog	d–						
13. candy	–d–						
14. table	t–						
15. apple	–p–						
Total							

Tabulated by:_____

INDIVIDUAL RECORD SHEET
Cerebral Palsy
Part Test B. Consonants

Name_____ Institution_____ Date_____

		Correct	Substitution	Omitted	Distorted	Response	Neutral
1. dog	–g						
2. cat	k–						
3. bathe	–ð						
4. foot	f–						
5. gun	g–						
6. sugar	–g–						
7. basket	–k–						
8. very	v–						
9. knife	–f						

*When the subject responds with a sound pattern which does not resemble the stimulus word in any respect, it is classed as neutral.

10. seven	−v−					
11. that	ð−					
12. thin	ө−					
13. father	−ð−					
14. Kathy	−ө−					
15. sofa	−f−					
16. stove	−v					
17. book	−k					
18. path	−ө					
Total						

Tabulated by:_____

INDIVIDUAL RECORD SHEET
Cerebral Palsy
Part Test C. Consonants

Name_____ Institution_____ Date_____

		Correct	Substi- tution	Omitted	Dis- torted	No Re- sponse	Neutral
1. car	−r						
2. leg	l−						
3. dish	−ʃ						
4. so	s−						
5. red	r−						
6. carry	−r−						
7. hello	−l−						
8. zoo	z−						
9. us	−s						
10. easy	−z−						
11. she	ʃ−						
12. fishes	−ʃ−						
13. usual	−ʒ−						
14. lesson	−s−						
15. has	−z						
16. ball	−l						
17. garage	−ʒ						
Total							

Tabulated by:_____

INDIVIDUAL RECORD SHEET
Cerebral Palsy
Part Test D. Consonants

Name_____ Institution_____ Date_____

		Correct	Substi- tuted	Omitted	Dis- torted	No Re- sponse	Neutral
1. ring	−ŋ						
2. chair	tʃ−						

3. age	−dʒ							
4. we	w−							
5. finger	−ŋ−							
6. teacher	−tʃ−							
7. why	ʍ−							
8. pigeon	−dʒ−							
9. nowhere	−ʍ−							
10. you	j−							
11. not	n−							
12. onion	−j−							
13. sunny	−n−							
14. awake	−w−							
15. much	−tʃ							
16. on	−n							
17. jack	dʒ−							
Total								

Tabulated by:_____

INDIVIDUAL RECORD SHEET
Cerebral Palsy
Part Test D. Vowels

Name_____ Institution_____ Date_____

		Correct	Substi-tuted	Omitted	Diph-thong-ized	Dis-torted	No Re-sponse	Neutral
1. bean	−i−							
2. Ed	ɛ−							
3. cook	−ʊ−							
4. eat	i−							
5. can	−æ−							
6. bed	−ɛ−							
7. up	ʌ−							
8. all	ɔ−							
9. coke	−o−							
10. in	ɪ−							
11. did	−ɪ−							
12. cut	−ʌ−							
13. oak	o−							
14. at	æ−							
15. moon	−u−							
16. ball	−ɔ−							
17. doll	−ɑ−							
18. on	ɑ−							
19. ooze	u−							
20. bird	−ɝ−							
Total								

Tabulated by:_____

INDIVIDUAL RECORD SHEET

Cerebral Palsy

Alternate Part Test A. Consonants

Name_____ Institution_____ Date_____

		Correct	Substi-tuted	Omitted	Dis-torted	No Re-sponse	Neutral
1. boy	b–						
2. bird	–d						
3. baby	–b–						
4. club	–b						
5. soup	–p						
6. comb	–m						
7. man	m–						
8. pie	p–						
9. coat	–t						
10. mammal	–m–						
11. butter	–t–						
12. duck	d–						
13. candle	–d–						
14. tree	t–						
15. puppy	–p–						
Total							

Tabulated by:_____

INDIVIDUAL RECORD SHEET

Cerebral Palsy

Alternate Part Test B. Consonants

Name_____ Institution_____ Date_____

		Correct	Substi-tuted	Omitted	Dis-torted	No Re-sponse	Neutral
1. pig	–g						
2. cow	k–						
3. breathe	–ɵ						
4. face	f–						
5. girl	g–						
6. cigar	–g̱						
7. biscuit	–k–						
8. vase	v–						
9. wife	–f						
10. clover	–v–						
11. them	ð–						
12. thumb	ɵ–						
13. mother	–ð–						
14. bathtub	–ɵ–						
15. rifle	–f						
16. serve	–v						

17. coke	−k						
18. teeth	−θ						
Total							

Tabulated by:_____

INDIVIDUAL RECORD SHEET
Cerebral Palsy
Alternate Part Test C. Consonants

		Correct	Substi-tuted	Omitted	Dis-torted	No Re-sponse	Neutral
1. far	−r						
2. like	l−						
3. fish	−ʃ						
4. sat	s−						
5. rib	r−						
6. ferry	−r						
7. solid	−l−						
8. zip	z−						
9. miss	−s						
10. daisy	−z−						
11. shut	ʃ−						
12. ashes	−ʃ−						
13. vision	−ʒ−						
14. essay	−s−						
15. his	−z						
16. fall	−l						
17. rouge	−ʒ						
Total							

Tabulated by:_____

INDIVIDUAL RECORD SHEET
Cerebral Palsy
Alternate Part Test D. Consonants

Name_____ Institution_____ Date_____

		Correct	Substi-tuted	Omitted	Dis-torted	No Re-sponse	Neutral
1. long	−ŋ						
2. chew	tʃ−						
3. page	−dʒ						
4. wash	w−						
5. singer	−ŋ−						
6. kitchen	−tʃ−						
7. when	ʍ−						
8. magic	−dj−						
9. awhile	−ʍ−						
10. yell	j−						

11. not   n–   _____ _____ _____ _____ _____
12. value   –l–   _____ _____ _____ _____ _____
13. funny   –n–   _____ _____ _____ _____ _____
14. reward   –w–   _____ _____ _____ _____ _____
15. rich   –tʃ   _____ _____ _____ _____ _____
16. ran   –n   _____ _____ _____ _____ _____
17. jug   dj–   _____ _____ _____ _____ _____
Total   _____ _____ _____ _____ _____

Tabulated by:_____

INDIVIDUAL RECORD SHEET
Cerebral Palsy
Alternate Part Test E. Vowels

Name_____ Institution_____ Date_____

		Correct	Substi-tuted	Omitted	Dis-torted	No Re-sponse	Neutral
1. elm	ɛ–						
2. oodles	u–						
3. it	I–						
4. book	–u–						
5. pet	–ɛ–						
6. bead	–i–						
7. add	æ–						
8. gun	–ʌ–						
9. auto	ɔ–						
10. tin	–I–						
11. bomb	–ɑ–						
12. spoon	–u–						
13. under	ʌ–						
14. old	o–						
15. olive	ɑ–						
16. eel	i–						
17. note	–o–						
18. cat	–æ–						
19. tall	–ɔ–						
20. hurt	–ɝ–						
Total							

Tabulated by:_____

PART X
BIBLIOGRAPHY

Bibliography

Adkins, Dorothy: *Construction and Analysis of Achievement Tests.* Washington, D. C., U. S. Government Printing Office, 1947.

Anastasi, Anne: *Psychological Testing.* New York, Macmillan, 1968.

Bangs, J. L.: A clinical analysis of the articulation defects in the feeble-minded. *J Speech Hearing Dis, 7*:343–356, 1942.

Barnes, H. G.: A diagnosis of the speech needs and abilities of students in a required course in speech training. Ph.D. dissertation, State University, Iowa, 1932.

Bartlett, M. S.: *J Roy Stat Soc (supple.), 4*:137, 1937.

Bottenberg, R. A., and Ward, J. H.: *Applied Linear Regression.* Personnel Research Laboratory, Aerospace Medical Division, Lockland Air Force Base, Texas. Technical Documentary Report PRLTDR–63–6. March, 1963.

Carnap, R.: *The Logical Syntax of Language.* London, Kegan, Paul, Trench, Trubner & Co., Ltd., 1937.

Castaneda, A., McCandless, B. R., and Palermo, D. S.: The children's form of the manifest anxiety scale. *Child Develop, 27 (No. 3).*

Chomsky, N.: Current issues in linguistic theory. In Foder, Jerry A., and Katz, Jerrold J. (Ed.) : *The Structure of Language.* Englewood, Prentice-Hall, 1964.

Cochran, W. G., and Cox G. M.: *Experimental Designs.* New York, John Wiley & Sons, 1953.

Cruickshank, W. M., and Raus, G. M.: *Cerebral Palsy: Its Individual and Community Problems.* Syracuse, Syracuse University Press, 1955.

Curtis, James T.: Disorders of voice. Ch. 4 in Johnson, Brown, Curtis, Edney and Keaster: *Speech Handicapped School Children.* New York, Harper, 1948.

DeLaguna, Grace Andrus: *Speech: Its Function and Development.* New Haven, Yale University Press, 1927.

Dunn, Lloyd M.: *Peabody Picture Vocabulary Test.* Minneapolis, American Guidance Service, 1959.

Fairbanks, Grant: *Voice and Articulation Drillbook.* Harper, New York, 1940.

Festinger, L.: Analysis of methods of calculating percent agreement. Unpublished memorandum, 1944.

Flanagan, J. C.: General considerations in the selection of test items and a short method of estimating the product-moment coefficient from data at the tails of the distribution. *J. Educ Psychol, 30*:674–680, 1939.

Flores, Pura M., and Irwin, Orvis C.: Status of five front consonants in the speech of cerebral palsy children. *J Speech Hearing Disorders, No. 21:* 238–244, 1956.

Fries, Charles C.: *The Structure of English: An Introduction to the Construction of English Sentences.* New York, Harcourt Brace & Co., 1952.

Gleason, H. A.: *Introduction to Descriptive Linguistics.* New York, Holt, Rinehart & Winston, 1961.

Hall, M. E.: Auditory factors in functional articulatory speech defects. *J Exper Educ, No. 7:*110–132, 1938.

Hammill, Don D., and Irwin, Orvis C.: Relations among measures of language of cerebral palsied and mentally retarded children. *Cerebral Palsy J, 27 (No. 1):* 10–12, 1965.

Hammill, Don D., and Irwin, Orvis C.: An abstraction test adapted for use with mentally retarded children. *Cerebral Palsy J, 27(No. 1):*8–9, 1965.

Hartley, R. V. L.: Transmission of information. *Bell System Tech J,* 1928.

Hays, William L.: *Statistics for Psychologists.* New York, Holt, Rinehart & Winston, 1963.

Heber, A.: A manual on terminology and classification in mental retardation. *Amer J Ment Defic (Monogr. Supple.),* 55–64, 1961b.

Hoyt, C.: Test reliability estimated by analysis of variance. *Psychometrica,* 6:153–60, 1941.

Irwin, Dale O.: Articulation of difficult speech sounds by two groups of retarded children. *Cerebral Palsy J, 27(No. 2):*3–7, 1966.

Irwin Orvis C.: Number and length of sentences in the language of mentally retarded children. *Cerebral Palsy J, 29(No. 1):*13–14, 1968.

Irwin Orvis C.: Correct status of vowels and consonants in the speech of children with cerebral palsy as measured by an integrated test. *Cerebral Palsy J, 29(No. 1):*9–12, 1968.

Irwin, Orvis C.: Relations among measures of the immediate memory span of retarded children. Unpublished study, 1968.

Irwin, Orvis C.: A manifest anxiety scale for use with cerebral palsied children. Unpublished study, 1968.

Irwin, Orvis C.: Cognitive trends in mentally retarded children. In Haywood, H. Carl (Ed.) : *Proceedings of the Peabody N.I.M.H. Conference on Social-Cultural Aspects of Mental Retardation.* New York, Appleton-Century-Crofts, 1970.

Irwin, Orvis C.: The nature of science. *Cerebral Palsy J, 29(No. 1):*4–9, 1968.

Irwin, Orvis C., and Korst, Joseph W.: Comparison of scores of cerebral palsied subnormal and normal children on five speech tests. *Cerebral Palsy J, 28(No. 3):*10–11, 1968.

Irwin, Orvis C., and Korst, Joseph W.: Correlations among five speech tests and the Wisc verbal scale. *Cerebral Palsy J, 28(No. 5):*9–11, 1967.

Irwin, Orvis C., and Korst, Joseph W.: A further study of the number and length of sentences in the language of cerebral palsied children. *Cerebral Palsy J, 28(No. 5):*3–4, 1967.

Irwin, Orvis C., and Korst, Joseph W.: Summary of reliability coefficients of six speech tests for use with handicapped children. *Cerebral Palsy J, 28 (No. 4)*:6–7, 1967.

Irwin, Orvis C., and Korst, Joseph W.: Comparison of scores of cerebral palsied, subnormal and normal children on five speech tests. *Cerebral Palsy J, 28(No. 3)*:10–11, 1967.

Irwin, Orvis C., and Hammill, Don D.: Effect of type of mental retardation on three language measures. *Cerebral Palsy J, 27(No. 1)*:9–10, 1966.

Irwin, Orvis C., and Hammill, Don D.: Effect of type, extent and degree of cerebral palsy on three measures of language. *Cerebral Palsy J, 26(No. 6)*: 7–9, 1965.

Irwin, Orvis C., and Hammill, Don D.: Regional and sex differences in the language of cerebral palsied children. *Cerebral Palsy J, 26(No. 5)*:11–12, 1965.

Irwin, Orvis C., and Hammill, Don D.: An item analysis of a sound discrimination test, Form A, for use with mentally retarded children. *Cerebral Palsy J, 26(No. 4)*:9–11, 1965.

Irwin, Orvis C., and Hammill, Don D.: A second comparison of sound discrimination of cerebral palsied and mentally retarded children. *Cerebral Palsy J, 26(No. 2)*:3–6, 1965.

Irwin, Orvis C., and Hammill, Don D.: A comparison of sound discrimination of mentally retarded and cerebral palsied children, Form A. *Cerebral Palsy Review, 26(No. 1)*:3–6, 1965.

Irwin, Orvis C., and Hammill, Don D.: Some results with an abstraction test with cerebral palsy children. *Cerebral Palsy Review, 25(No. 5)*:10–11, 1964 (b).

Irwin, Orvis C., and Hammill, Don D.: An abstraction test for use with cerebral palsied children. *Cerebral Palsy Review, 25(No. 4)*:3–9, 1964 (a).

Irwin, Orvis C., and Jensen, Paul J.: A third study of a sound discrimination test for use with cerebral palsied children. *Cerebral Palsy Review, 25(No. 1)*:3–7, 1964.

Irwin, Orvis C., and Jensen, Paul J.: A parallel test of sound discrimination for use with cerebral palsied children, Form B. *Cerebral Palsy Review, 24(No. 5)*:3–10, 1963.

Irwin, Orvis C., and Jensen, Paul J.: A test of sound discrimination for use with cerebral palsied children. *Cerebral Palsy Review, 24(No. 3)*:3–7, 1963.

Irwin, Orvis C., and Jensen, Paul J.: A test of sound discrimination for use with cerebral palsied children, Form A. *Cerebral Palsy Review, 24(No. 4)*:5–11, 1963.

Irwin, Orvis C.: Replications and reliabilities of four speech tests. *Cerebral Palsy J, 28(No. 3)*:5–6, 1967.

Irwin, Orvis C.: Number and length of sentences in the language of mentally retarded children. *Cerebral Palsy J, 28(No. 1)*:9–10, 1967.

Irwin, Orvis C.: A comparison of the vocabulary of use and of understanding by mentally retarded children. *Cerebral Palsy J, 27(No. 6)*:8–10, 1966.

Irwin, Orvis C.: Length of declarative sentences in the language of cerebral palsied children. *Cerebral Palsy J, 27(No. 6):*4–5, 1966.

Irwin, Orvis C.: A language test for use with cerebral palsied children. *Cerebral Palsy J, 27(No. 5):*6–8, 1966.

Irwin, Orvis C., The relation of vocabularies of use and understanding by cerebral palsied children to several variables. *Cerebral Palsy J, 27(No. 4):* 3–4, 1966.

Irwin, Orvis C.: Vocabulary ability of two samples of cerebral palsied children. *Cerebral Palsy J, 27(No. 3):*14–15, 1966.

Irwin, Orvis C.: A comparison of the vocabulary of use and of understanding of cerebral palsied children. *Cerebral Palsy J, 27(No. 3):*7–11, 1966.

Irwin, Dale O.: Reliability of the Wechsler Intelligence Scale for children. *J Educ. Measurement, 3(No. 4):*287–292, 1966.

Irwin, Orvis C.: A note on the comparison of articulation of children with cerebral palsy who were given mental tests and those who were not. *Cerebral Palsy Review, 24(No. 2):*5–6, 1963.

Irwin, Orvis C.: Applicability of an articulation test with mentally retarded children. *Cerebral Palsy Review, 24(No. 1):*3–8, 1963.

Irwin, Orvis C.: Substitutions and omissions of initial consonant blends in the speech of children with cerebral palsy. *Cerebral Palsy Review, 23(No. 5):*5–6, 1962.

Irwin, Orvis C.: Status of articulation of final reversed consonant blends by children with cerebral palsy. *Cerebral Palsy Review, 23(No. 2):*17–19, 1962.

Irwin, Orvis C.: A second comparative study of articulation of children with cerebral palsy and of mentally retarded children. *Cerebral Palsy Review, 23(No. 1):*17–19, 1962.

Irwin, Orvis C.: A test of triple consonant blends for use with children with cerebral palsy. *Cerebral Palsy Review, 23(No. 4):*9–11, 1963.

Irwin, Orvis C.: Standardization of a test of final double reversed consonant blends for use with children with cerebral palsy. *Cerebral Palsy Review, 22(No. 4):*21–24, 1961.

Irwin, Orvis C.: Difficulties of consonant sounds in terms of manner and place of articulation and of voicing in the speech of cerebral palsied children. *Cerebral Palsy Review, 24(No. 3):*13–16, 1961.

Irwin, Orvis C.: Correct status of diphthongs in the speech of children with cerebral palsy. *Cerebral Palsy Review, 22(No. 1):*6–7, 1961.

Irwin, Orvis C.: Difficulties of consonant and vowel sounds in the speech of children with cerebral palsy. *Cerebral Palsy Review, 22(No. 5):*14–15, 1961.

Irwin, Orvis C.: Verification of results obtained with an integrated articulation test for use with children with cerebral palsy. *Cerebral Palsy Review, 22(No. 5):*8–13, 1961.

Irwin, Orvis C.: A manual of articulation testing for use with children with cerebral palsy. *Cerebral Palsy Review, 22(No. 3):*1–20, 1961.

Irwin, Orvis C.: Correct status of vowels and consonants in the speech of cerebral palsied children as measured by an integrated test. *Cerebral Palsy Review, 22(No. 2):*21–24, 1961.

Irwin, Orvis C.: Comparison of articulation scores of children with cerebral palsy and mentally retarded children. *Cerebral Palsy Review, 22(No. 2)*: 1–2, 1961.

Irwin, Orvis C.: A short articulation test of ten consonants for use with children with cerebral palsy. *Cerebral Palsy Review, 22(No. 2)*:28–31, 1961.

Irwin, Orvis C.: Correct status of vowels in the speech of children with cerebral palsy. *Cerebral Palsy Review, 21(No. 5)*:10–11, 1960.

Irwin, Orvis C.: Correct articulation of ten difficult consonants by children with cerebral palsy. *Cerebral Palsy Review, 21(No. 1)*:6–7, 1960.

Irwin, Orvis C.: A short vowel test for use with children with cerebral palsy. *Cerebral Palsy Review, 21(No. 4)*:3–4, 1960.

Irwin, Orvis C.: Language and Communication. Ch. 12 in Mussen's *Handbook of Research in Child Development*. New York, John Wiley & Sons, 1960.

Irwin, Orvis C.: Correct status of final double consonant blends in the speech of children with cerebral palsy. *Cerebral Palsy Review, 20(No. 3)*:10–12, 1959.

Irwin, Orvis C.: A sixth short consonant test for use with cerebral palsied children. *Cerebral Palsy Review, 20(No. 2)*:13–16, 1959.

Irwin, Orvis C.: Substitution and omissions of initial double consonant blends in the speech of children with cerebral palsy. *Cerebral Palsy Review, 20(No. 3)*:10–12, 1959.

Irwin, Orvis C.: A fifth short consonant test for use with children with cerebral palsy. *Cerebral Palsy Review, 20(No. 1)*:7–9, 1959.

Irwin, Orvis C.: A fourth short consonant test for use with children with cerebral palsy. *Cerebral Palsy Review, 19*:15–16, 1959.

Irwin, Orvis C.: A third short consonant test for use with children with cerebral palsy. *Cerebral Palsy Review, 19(No. 1)*:8–10, 1958.

Irwin, Orvis C.: Correct status of initial double consonant blends in the speech of children with cerebral palsy. *Cerebral Palsy Review, 19(No. 6)*: 9–13, 1958.

Irwin, Orvis C.: Phonetical description of speech development in childhood. Ch. 25 in Kaiser's *Manual of Phonetics*. Amsterdam, North Holland Publishing Co., 1957.

Irwin, Orvis C.: Correct status of a set of six consonants in the speech of children with cerebral palsy. *Cerebral Palsy Review, 17(No. 6)*:148–150, 1956.

Irwin, Orvis C.: Validation of short consonant articulation tests for use with cerebral palsied children. *Cerebral Palsy Review. 18(No. 2)*:12, 1957.

Irwin, Orvis C.: Correct status of a third set of consonants in the speech of cerebral palsy children. *Cerebral Palsy Review, 18(No. 3)*:17–20, 1957.

Irwin, Orvis C.: A second short test for use with cerebral palsied children. *Cerebral Palsy Review, 18(No. 4)*:18–19, 1957.

Irwin, Orvis C.: A second study of substitution and omission errors in the speech of children with cerebral palsy. *Cerebral Palsy Review, 17(No. 4):* 109, 1956.

Irwin, Orvis C.: Substitution and omission errors in the speech of children who have cerebral palsy. *Cerebral Palsy Review, 17(No. 3):*75, 1956.

Irwin, Orvis C.: A short test of five consonants for use with cerebral palsy children. *J Speech Hearing Dis, 21(No. 4):*446–449, 1956.

Irwin, Orvis C., and Thayer, Curry: Vowel elements in the crying vocalization of infants under ten days of age. *Child Develop, 12:*99–109, 1941.

Karlin, I. W., and Strazzula, M.: Speech and language problems of mentally deficient children. *J Speech Hearing Dis, 17:*286–294, 1952.

Kenyon, J. S., and Knott, T. A.: *A Progressive Pronouncing Dictionary of American English.* Springfield, (Mass.) , G. & C. Merriam, 1951.

Kerlinger, Fred N.: *Foundations of Behavioral Research.* New York, Holt, Rinehart & Winston, 1965.

Korst, Joseph W., and Irwin, Orvis C.: Verbal and numerical immediate memory spans of mentally retarded children. *Cerebral Palsy J, 29(No. 4):* 1–4, 1968.

Korst, Joseph W., and Irwin, Orvis C.: Immediate memory span of mentally retarded children. *Cerebral Palsy J, 29(No. 3):*10–11, 1968.

Kuder, G. F., and Richardson, M. N.: The theory of the estimation of test reliability. *Psychomentric, No. 2:*151–160, 1937.

Lindquist, E. F.: Goodness of fit of trend curves and significance of trend differences. Psychometrica, *121(No. 2):*65–78, 1947.

Lindquist, E. F. (Ed.) : *Educational Measurement.* Washington, D. C., American Council of Education, 1951.

Lindquist, E. F.: Design and Analysis of Experiments in Psychology and Education. Boston, Houghton Mifflin, 1953.

Margenau, Henry: *The Nature of Physical Reality.* New York, McGraw-Hill, 1950.

McCurry, William H., and Irwin, Orvis C.: A study of word approximations in the spontaneous speech of infants. *J Speech Hearing Dis, 18:*133–139, 1953.

Norton, Dee W.: An empirical investigation of the effects on non-normality and heterogeneity upon the F-test of analysis of variance. Ph.D. thesis State University, Iowa, 1952.

Powers, Margaret Hall: Functional disorders of articulation. In *Handbook of Speech Disorders.* Translated by L. E. (Ed.) . New York, Appleton-Century-Crofts, 1957.

Roe, Vivian, and Milisen, Robert: The effect of maturation upon defective articulation in elementary grades. *J Speech Hearing Dis, 7:*37–50, 1942.

Rutherford, Bernice R.: Frequency of articulation substitutions handicapped by cerebral palsy. *J Speech Hearing Dis, No. 4:*285–287, 1939.

Sayer, H. K.: The effect of maturation upon defective articulation in grades seven through twelve. *J Speech Hearing Dis, 14:*202–227, 1940.

Spriesterbach, D. C., Darley, F. L., and Rouse, V.: Articulation of a group of children with cleft lips and palates. *J Speech Hearing Dis, 4:*436–445, 1956.

Templin, Mildren: *Certain Language Skills in Children.* Minneapolis, University of Minneapolis, 1957.

Terman, L. M., and Merrill, M. A.: *Stanford-Binet Intelligence Scale.* Boston, Houghton Mifflin Co., 1960.

Torgerson, Warren S.: *Theory and Methods of Scaling.* New York, John Wiley & Sons, 1958.

United Cerebral Palsy: *Proceedings of the Activities of Tenth Annual United Cerebral Palsy Workshop.* Austin, University of Texas, 1962.

Utley, J.: *What's its name?* Urbana, University of Illinois Press, 1950.

Van Riper, C.: *Speech Correction Principles and Methods* (2nd ed). New York, Prentice-Hall, 1947.

Walker, H. M., and Lev, J.: *Statistical Inference.* New York, Henry Holt & Co., 1953.

Wechsler, D.: *Intelligence Scale for Children.* New York, Psychological Corp., 1959.

Wellman, Beth L., Case, Ida Mae, Mengert, Ida Goarder, and Bradbury, Dorothy E.: *Speech Sounds of Young Children.* University of Iowa Study of Child Welfare, Vol. 5 (No. 2), Iowa City, University of Iowa Press, 1931.

Westlake, Harold: Muscle training for cerebral palsy speech cases. *J Speech Hearing Dis, 16:*103–109, 1951.

Whorf, B. L.: *Four Articles on Metalinguistics.* Washington. Foreign Service Institute, 1950.

Winer, B. J.: *Statistical Principles in Experimental Design.* New York, McGraw-Hill, 1962.

Wundt, B. L.: *Völkerpsychologic.* Vol. 1, *Die Sprache.* Leipzig, Engelmann, 1900.

AUTHOR INDEX

Adkins, D., XVIII, 22, 104
Anastasi, A., XVIII, 22, 104

Bartlett, M., 44, 45, 49, 59
Bangs, J., 130
Bradbury, D., 16

Carnap, R., 269
Case, I., 16
Castaneda, A., 265
Chomsky, N., XI, 269
Cochran, W., 59, 71, 132, 143, 174
Cox, G., 59, 71, 132, 143, 174

Darley, F., 130
DeLaguna, G., 269

Fairbanks, G., 5, 130
Festinger, L., 211
Flanagan, J., XVI, 26, 35
Flores, P., 10
Fries, C., 237

Gleason, H., XI

Hammill, D., 95, 177, 191, 200, 287
Hartley, R., 269
Heber, A., 241
Hoyt, C., 6, 19, 25, 35

Irwin, D., 129, 140, 142, 144
Irwin, O., 211, 249

Jakobson, R. and Halle, M., XI
Jensen, P., 159

Karlin, J., 130
Kenyon, J., 12, 211
Kerlinger, F., XIII
Knott, T., 12, 211
Korst, J., 249, 252, 279, 283, 290

Kuder, G., XVIII, 5, 6, 18, 25, 38, 41, 52, 55, 66, 77, 79, 85, 87, 102, 124, 136, 146, 163, 169, 176, 185, 187, 197, 199, 280, 295, 297, 300, 302

Margenau, H., IX, XII, 313
McCandless, B., 265
McCurry, W., 211
Merrill, M., 249
Milisen, R., 130

Palermo, D., 265
Powers, M., 130

Richardson, M., XVIII, 5, 6, 18, 25, 38, 41, 52, 55, 66, 67, 79, 85, 87, 102, 124, 136, 141, 163, 169, 176, 185, 187, 197, 199, 280, 295, 300, 302
Roe, V., 130
Rouse, V., 130

Saylor, H., 130
Schwarz, R., 160
Spriesterbach, D., 130
Strazzula, M., 130

Templin, M., 37, 46, 48, 51, 52, 55, 56, 57, 62, 66, 69, 73, 74, 76, 178, 179, 182, 217
Terman, L., 249
Torgerson, W., XIII

Utley, J., 10

Van Riper, C., 130

Wechsler, D., 186, 249, 261
Wellman, B., 16
Westlake, H., 28, 32
Whorf, B., 269
Wundt, B., 269

367

SUBJECT INDEX

A

Administration, of tests, xix, 11, 142, 195
Abstraction, definition of, 191

C

CA, 31-32, 42-43, 54-55, 70, 81, 89, 97, 105,
127, 133, 142, 167, 174, 178, 180, 201,
206, 212, 219, 229, 250, 256, 260, 295,
302, 304, 306
Communication, social definition, xii
Comparison
of CPs and MRs, 146, 151, 177, 206,
231, 244
of degree of CP, 97
of type of CP, 97
Computer, 96
Connectibility, xiv
Consonant, definition of, 112, 113
Construct
operational, xiv, 313
constitutive, xiv, 313
Correct scores, 12, 13, 16, 32, 49, 62, 72,
83, 93, 147, 153, 212
Correlations of scores
with the PPVT, 285
with the Wisc, 285
Criteria, of test usefulness, 5

D

Degrees of MR, 187
Diagnoses, medical, 44-45, 58, 70-71, 82,
90, 103, 143, 165, 168, 174, 175, 201,
225, 274, 295, 302, 303, 310
Difficulty, xvi, 6-7, 19-20, 26, 35, 38, 53,
67, 75, 78, 86, 109-111, 112-122, 125,
133, 139, 161, 171-172, 181, 193, 194,
204, 296, 302
Discriminating power, xvi, 7, 20, 26, 35,
38, 54, 68, 75, 79, 86, 125, 126, 161, 171-
172, 193, 194, 204, 302
Discription of subjects, appendix, 319-336

E

Educables, 132, 170
Errors, 16-17, 49-50, 62-64, 71-72, 76, 82,
93, 133, 148, 153, 310, 311
Extreme groups method, 22

F

Formulas
Bartlett, 45, 49
Cochran-Cox, 59, 132, 143
Festinger, 211
Flanagan, 186
Hoyt, 6, 25, 280
Kuder-Richardson, 25, 38, 52, 66, 85,
102, 124, 163, 280, 297

H

Hemiplegia, 58-59, 71, 89, 104, 143, 295,
310

I

Information theory, xiv
Instructions
to examiner, 194-195
to subject, 215
Integrated test, 99-108
Intercorrelations, of speech tests, 284
Involvement, degree of, 30-31, 46, 59-60,
96, 97, 103, 200, 222, 225, 274-275, 295,
302
Involvement, extent of, 45, 59, 71, 82, 90,
103, 144, 168, 175, 200, 225, 295, 302
Item analysis, xvi-xvii
IQ, 31, 60, 70, 81, 89, 105, 127, 133, 142,
167, 174, 180, 206, 220, 254, 295

M

MA, 43, 55, 70, 81, 89, 105, 127, 133, 142,
167, 174, 201, 220, 230, 251, 255, 257,
295, 302, 304, 306
Meaning, xiii, xiv
Memory span

and chronological age, 256
and mental age, 254

N

Neutral, 12

O

Operations, xv
Oral function, 32
Order, 12, 13, 311
Organization, of topics, xx

P

Pearson, coefficient of correlation, 303
Picture test, description of, 214
Position, 12, 14, 30, 82, 83, 90, 102, 105, 112-119, 132, 143, 168, 175, 295, 300
Profiles, 112-122
Pronouncing dictionary, Kenyon and Knott, 211

R

Rating, speech, 46, 104, 174, 201, 275
Ratio, of two vocabularies, 221, 231
Regions, 49, 62, 69, 70, 92, 159-160, 170, 184, 196, 204, 288, 289
Reliability, xvii-xviii
of observer, xvi
of test, xviii, 6, 18-19, 25, 29, 35, 38, 52, 57, 66, 77, 85, 102, 124, 131, 136-137, 160, 163, 172-173, 178, 185, 195, 197, 205, 217, 228, 272, 277-278, 280, 281, 295, 296, 297, 300, 301, 302, 305, 307
Respiratory function, 32

S

Sentence
complete, 287
incomplete, 287
Sex, 29, 43-44, 70, 73, 81, 83, 89, 101, 131-132, 159-160, 170, 177, 184, 196, 204, 218, 229, 238, 239, 242, 243, 254, 256, 258, 272, 288, 289, 306
Short tests, 5, 18, 25, 34, 52, 66, 73, 77, 85, 129
Speech, parts of, 219
Stimulation, 12
Structural linguists, xiv

T

Tests, of
abstraction, 191, 344-345
articulation, 99, 129, 339, 340-342
immediate memory span, 252, 345
language, 215, 216, 271
manifest anxiety, 265, 346
sound discrimination, 159, 170, 343-344
vocabulary, 214
Theory, x-xiv, 313-314
Trainables, 132, 170
Trends, age, 230

V

Validity, xviii, 22-24, 26-27, 36, 39, 52, 66-67, 74, 78, 85, 104-105, 124, 137-138, 164, 173-174, 178, 186-187, 197-198, 205, 272, 296, 298, 301, 302
Variables, articulation, sound discrimination, abstraction, vocabularies, immediate memory span, manifest anxiety, ix

U

Uniqueness, xvi, 8, 20, 26, 36, 39, 54, 68, 75, 79, 87, 125, 140, 161, 171-172, 193, 194, 204, 296, 302

W

Word approximation, definition of, 211